Thomas Hall

Full Report of the Trial of Thomas Hall

For the Murder of Captain Henry Cain

Thomas Hall

Full Report of the Trial of Thomas Hall
For the Murder of Captain Henry Cain

ISBN/EAN: 9783337091040

Printed in Europe, USA, Canada, Australia, Japan

Cover: Foto ©ninafisch / pixelio.de

More available books at **www.hansebooks.com**

FULL REPORT

OF THE

TRIAL OF THOMAS HALL

FOR THE MURDER OF

CAPTAIN HENRY CAIN.

Before His Honor Mr. JUSTICE WILLIAMS, at the Supreme Court, Dunedin, January, 1887.

REPRINTED FROM THE "OTAGO DAILY TIMES."

Dunedin:
PRINTED AT THE "OTAGO DAILY TIMES" OFFICE, HIGH STREET.

MDCCCLXXXVII.

THE TIMARU MURDER CASE.

TRIAL AT DUNEDIN OF THOMAS HALL FOR THE MURDER OF CAPTAIN CAIN.

FRIDAY, JANUARY 21, 1887.

(Before his Honor Mr Justice Williams.)

THE GRAND JURY.

The following gentlemen comprised the grand jury:—Messrs George M. Barr (foreman), William G. Neill, John W. Paulin, George Edmund Dermer, Maurice Joel, John Hislop, John Gillies, James Durston, France Arthur Cutten, Thomas Cullen, Henry Crust, Daniel Catchpole, Duncan Campbell, John Brown, George Blyth, Charles Frederick Black, and David Baxter.

HIS HONOR'S CHARGE.

His Honor delivered the following charge to the grand jury:—

Mr Foreman and gentlemen of the grand jury,—I have asked you to come together again to consider a charge of murder. I do not propose to discuss the evidence at any length. I shall confine myself to pointing out the salient features of the case made against the accused by the depositions. The accused Thomas Hall is charged with the wilful murder of Henry Cain. Henry Cain died on the 29th January 1886. He had been ill some time before from dropsy and kidney disease. The doctors certify that he died from that cause. At the time of his death there was no suspicion of any foul play. Some months after his death suspicions arose, and the body was exhumed. In it was found antimony in a quantity sufficient in itself, according to the medical testimony, to have accelerated death in a person in the weak condition in which Cain was shortly before his death was. Now antimony is not naturally found in the human body, and is not a product of decomposition. If, then, as it must have been, by Cain in his lifetime, how was it administered? His medical man, Dr Macintyre, had on various occasions prescribed for him, but antimony never entered into any of those prescriptions. To account, therefore, for its presence there can be but three hypotheses: Firstly, that it was taken or administered by pure accident; secondly, that it was wilfully taken by Cain; and thirdly, that it was wilfully administered by someone else. You have to consider which of these the evidence shows as most probable. The evidence

further shows some grounds for supposing that more antimony was administered than was actually found in the body after death. During the latter part of his life Cain suffered from constant vomiting: a symptom, indeed, of his disease, but also a characteristic symptom of antimonial poisoning. He seems to have specially complained that whisky, which he had been in the habit of taking for many years, caused him to vomit. Two witnesses who took liquor in Cain's house speak of being sick immediately after, but, on the other hand, other witnesses who also took liquor suffered no ill effects. The medical testimony does not seem to have been very fully brought out at the preliminary inquiry, and possibly from the quantity of antimony found in the body, and from the appearance of the different organs, the doctors may be able to draw some further inferences material to the case. The accused Hall had married the step-daughter of the deceased in May 1885. The deceased objected to the marriage, and Hall and he were not at that time on friendly terms. About three months before Cain's decease, however, these differences were made up, and Hall became a daily visitor at the house, calling morning and evening and often dining with the deceased alone. It is suggested that the vomiting commenced, or at any rate became regular, shortly after the time Hall's visits commenced. In May 1885 Hall had purchased antimony and also a work on poisons, which he appears to have bought especially to ascertain the operation of this particular drug. The book contains the date "1882" in Hall's handwriting, suggesting that he then had it in his possession—a suggestion which was of course untrue. In August 1886 Hall was arrested on another charge—a charge of attempting to poison by antimony—and antimony was then found in his possession. He then admitted that he had purchased antimony, and stated that he had used it for a long time for cigarettes for asthma. For some time before Cain's death Hall had been in great financial difficulties, and had resorted to forgery to alleviate these difficulties. In several ways Cain's death would have been a direct or indirect pecuniary benefit to Hall. Cain's family consisted of two step-daughters, Mrs Hall and Mrs Newton. There is nothing to show that Hall knew how Cain had disposed of his property by his will,

4

but as a matter of fact the will, as might have been anticipated, gave the property between these two daughters. The value of Mrs Hall's share was about £250. There were also two deeds of settlement under which Mrs Hall had an interest. As to one of them, Mrs Hall and Mrs Newton, her sister, had an equal interest in the income of the fund. By a deed dated in December 1885 Mrs Hall and Mrs Newton had granted to Cain a life annuity of £300 a year and the use for life of the house where he resided and the grounds attached. By Cain's death half of this annuity and half the rental of the house would fall back to Mrs Hall. As to the other settlement, it was made by Mrs Hall, then Miss Espie, of her property apparently a considerable time before she married Hall. By that settlement she had put the *corpus* of her property out of her reach, and had vested it in Cain and Mr Le Cren upon trusts to pay her the income for her separate use. This settlement Hall wished to cancel, and suggested to LeCren a friendly suit for that purpose which should be undefended by the trustees. Mr Le Cren had no objection to these proceedings, but Mr Cain always objected to destroying the trust. Two days before Cain's death a suit was commenced by Hall on Mrs Hall's behalf, and in the following April Mr Le Cren paid Hall over £700, the amount of the trust moneys in hand. Cain's death, therefore, would apparently get rid of the obstacle in Hall's way to obtaining this money. The case, therefore, as disclosed by the depositions, is shortly this : Cain's death was accelerated by antimony. The hypothesis of its accidental administration or its having been wilfully taken by Cain is improbable. Hall had constant access to Cain. Hall had antimony in his possession, and had studied the subject of antimonial poison. Hall was urgently in want of money, and Cain's death would help to get him money. If you think three is *prima facie* evidence that Cain's death was accelerated, even in the smallest degree, by antimony wilfully administered by Hall, you should find a true bill. Gentlemen, if you will retire to your room the bill will be laid before you.

The grand jury retired at 20 minutes past 10 o'clock, and after deliberating for two hours and 20 minutes returned a true bill.

The court was then adjourned until 10 o'clock on Monday next.

MONDAY, JANUARY 24.

(Before his Honor Mr Justice Williams and a Special Jury.)

THE ARRAIGNMENT.

Thomas Hall was arraigned on Monday upon an indictment charging him that he, on the 9th January 1886, did feloniously, wilfully, and with malice aforethought, kill and murder one Henry Cain.

The prisoner pleaded " Not guilty."

Mr B. C. Haggitt (Crown prosecutor at Dunedin), assisted by Mr White (Crown prosecutor at Timaru), appeared for the Crown ; Mr F. R.

Chapman, with him Mr J. E. Denniston (instructed by Mr Perry, of Timaru) for the defence.

The following gentlemen were empanelled and sworn as a special jury :—William Henry Churton (foreman),Samuel Barningham, Robert Brownlie, John Campbell Morris, John M'Kay, James Williams, David Wishart, William Proudfoot Watson, Henry Allen, James Dow, William Asher, Charles M'Queen.

THE CROWN PROSECUTOR'S ADDRESS.

Mr Haggitt (the Crown prosecutor) opened the case for the Crown as follows :—May it please your honor and gentlemen of the jury. The indictment which has just been read to yon charges the prisoner with the willful murder of Henry Cain. Henry Cain was an old sea captain. He was known generally as Captain Cain or the captain, and resided at Timaru. His house was called Woodlands, and it was situated immediately outside the town of Timaru. He was a widower and had two stepdaughters—the one Mrs Newton and the other Mrs Hall, the wife of the prisoner. Mrs Newton was married first, and after her marriage Mrs Hall, the other stepdaughter, kept house for Cain up to the time of her marriage, which took place on the 26th of May 1885. After Mrs Hall's marriage Mrs Newton returned again to live with her stepfather, and continued to live with him—with the exception of two short intervals, during which she was absent on visits to her friends—from that time up to the time of his death, on the 20th of January 1886. At the time of the prisoner's marriage he and the late Captain Cain were not on good terms: in fact Cain was so much opposed to the marriage that he purposely absented himself from Timaru at the time it was to take place in order that he might not be present at the ceremony. Afterwards, however, he and the prisoner became reconciled, and shortly after Mrs Newton returned home from the last visit she paid before the captain's death—about the end of October—the prisoner became a frequent visitor at the house. At this time Captain Cain was in ill health. He was an old man, and he had had a severe illness some 18 months previously and had never entirely recovered his strength. He was suffering from kidney disease and dropsy, and had also suffered from chronic bronchitis, which necessitated him taking a considerable quantity of cough mixture. He was, however, still able to get about as usual ; he used to take a drive daily into Timaru, and still relished his meals and enjoyed his glass of whisky. But shortly after this time, and towards the end of November, his whisky began to disagree with him Several times after taking it he became violently sick, and ultimately he had to give it up altogether. Captain Cain was then advised to take brandy, and afterwards champagne, port wine, and claret in turns, but the sickness still continued at intervals down to the time of his death. He died, as I have already told you, on the morning of the 29th January 1886, and he was buried in the cemetery at Timaru two days afterwards. Dr Macintyre, a medical gentleman residing at Timaru, attended Captain Cain throughout his last illness. He attended him at intervals from July up to the 17th of December, and from the 17th December down to the day before he died he was constantly in attendance on him, and saw him daily. Dr Macintyre was somewhat surprised at the persistent vomiting and some other of the symptoms which developed themselves in the course of Captain Cain's illness, especially the diarrhœa, but he had no reason at that time to suspect any foul play, and at the time that Captain Cain died he had no idea that it was not the result of natural causes, and no suspicion was aroused at the time of his having been poisoned. Shortly after Captain Cain's death the prisoner and his wife took up their residence at Woodlands. In June Mrs Hall was confined. At this time, which as you will gather was some five months after Captain Cain's death, certain circumstances arose, the effect of which was to forcibly recall to Dr Macintyre the symptoms exhibited by Captain Cain during his last illness, and his suspicions were consequently aroused, and he caused such steps to be taken that the body of Captain Cain was exhumed on the 27th September 1886, just eight months after the time it had been buried. A *post mortem* was made by Dr Ogston and Dr Hogg, of Timaru, and the stomach, portions of the small and large intestines, the bladder, and portions of the liver, spleen, and kidneys, and some liquid from the chest and bladder, were put into bottles, which were corked and taken to Dunedin for analysis at the chemical laboratory at the University. On the same night that these were brought down an analysis was commenced by Dr Black, assisted by Dr Ogston and Dr Hogg, and the result of that analysis was to leave no doubt that antimony was present in large quantities in the body of Captain Cain. I may mention to you that the gentlemen who made the analysis looked for nothing else but antimony. You will hear presently that such symptoms as Captain Cain exhibited might have been caused by atropia, which is belladonna, or by colchicum; but these are vegetable poisons, and after the interval which had elapsed between the death of Captain Cain, and the exhumation of the body the analysts were of opinion that it was utterly useless to look for such poisons, as they disappear very rapidly; in fact, they disappear in a very much shorter time than elapsed since the body was buried, and they therefore decided that it was useless to look for these. We shall prove to you, gentlemen, that in the enfeebled condition Captain Cain was reduced for some short time before his death a very small quantity of antimony would have been sufficient to cause death, and that the administration of such irritants as I have mentioned—atropia, colchicum, or antimony—to a person in his condition would certainly have accelerated death. Now, gentlemen, the question which you will have to determine on this inquiry is how the antimony that was undoubtedly found in Captain Cain's body got there. We shall prove to you that it must have been administered to him during his lifetime, by some person, and I think, gentlemen,

the evidence will satisfy you that the person who administered it must have been the prisoner. Gentlemen, it is a maxim that if you wish to discover the author of any bad action, you should seek first to discover the person to whom the perpetration of that bad action would be advantageous. We shall show you that the prisoner had something to gain by the death of Captain Cain; in other words, that he had a motive for wishing for his death. We will then satisfy you that Hall had in his possession the means of accelerating Captain Cain's death, and that amongst other kinds of poison that he had the very kind of poison which was found in the body. Next we shall satisfy you that the prisoner had made the subject of poisoning generally a special study. We shall then show you that the prisoner had ample opportunities for administering the poisons to Captain Cain if so inclined, and that from the symptoms which were exhibited by Captain Cain in his lifetime he must have been made the receptacle of irritant poisons for more than a month before his death, in greater or less quantities, and at more or less frequent intervals; and lastly, gentlemen, I shall, I believe, be able to adduce to you evidence confirmatory of the result and the analysis; that is to say, evidence that similar symptoms were produced in another case.

Mr Chapman : This is the point, you honor, to which we object.

His Honor : Yes; that is the part of the evidence which it is contended is objectionable. There is no need to discuss the question of the admissibility of the evidence at this stage; it is enough that it can be questioned. The question can be raise afterwards.

Mr Haggitt : I submit that it cannot be questioned.

His Honor : We will not discuss that now. You will be kind enough to abide by my ruling.

Mr Haggitt; I do not wish to dispute your ruling, but at the same time—

His Honor : Very well, continue your address then.

Mr Haggitt : First, then, gentlemen, as to motive. We shall prove to you that the prisoner for some time before his marriage to Captain Cain's stepdaughter carried on business in partnership with a person named Meason, under the style of Hall and Meason, and that their business was that of landbrokers and surveyors, combined with a loan and discount business. They kept their account with the Bank of New South Wales at Timaru, and the prisoner managed and attended to the banking business of the partnership. . We shall prove to you that the firm was in great financial difficulties; that they had misappropriated trust moneys, and that in order to save their credit the prisoner had forged several promissory notes which he had got discounted by the bank, and which as they came due he retired by means of other forged notes, and in some instances he had forged mortgage securities.in the names of the makers of these notes in order to induce the bank to discount them and the renewals of them, and the more readily to induce the belief that they were genuine business transactions of the firm. In a word, gentlemen, we shall prove that the prisoner was hopelessly involved in financial difficulties, and had committed crimes which might any day be discovered, with the result that he would be disgraced, prosecuted, and punished. Now, gentlemen, this was the prisoner's position as far back as January 1885, and it got worse and worse before the end of that year. Before the accused married, which was on the 26th of May 1885, he had forged one promissory note for £800, and two months after his marriage we shall prove that he got his wife to make a will in his favour, leaving everything to him absolutely. In the following month he insured her life for £6000 with the Australian Mutual Provident Society.

Mr Chapman: I submit this is very wide of the mark as to motive.

His Honor: I do not see at present that this is relevant. It seems to be very doubtful whether that has anything to do with the case.

Mr Haggitt: We shall prove also that Mrs Hall was entitled to considerable sums of money and properties by certain wills and settlements which would only come into actual possession on Cain's death. Two of these settlements were made by Cain himself, the one in February 1870 and the other in July 1870. Under these settlements Mrs Hall would on Cain's death become entitled to properties worth several thousand pounds, including Woodlands, house and grounds, the residence of Captain Cain, and 40 acres of ground surrounding it, which alone was worth £6500. In this property you will find by a deed which was made in December 1885, Cain had a life interest, and he was besides entitled to an annuity of £300 a year out of the trust funds. By Cain's death, therefore, this property of Woodlands would be free of the life interest, and the annuity, of course, would cease; so that you will see that a considerable pecuniary advantage from this source alone would result to Mrs Hall, and therefore to the prisoner from the death of Captain Cain. I do not propose, gentlemen, to take up your time by mentioning now in detail all the pecuniary advantages that would accrue to the prisoner from Cain's death—they will come out by-and-bye in the evidence; but I may mention here that Cain had property of his own irrespective of this trust property, and that property of course he could dispose of by his will, and I submit to you that as his two stepdaughters were his nearest connections, and were always with him, it is reasonable to suppose that prisoner would calculate on his wife getting her share of anything that Captain Cain might leave. That he did calculate on getting something by the death of Captain Cain there will be some evidence before you, as we shall prove that in January 1886—shortly before Captain Cain's death, and when the prisoner was on good terms with him, and constantly in his company—he was told by his wife that Cain had made a new will, and he was apparently very much pleased with the intelligence, and said to his wife "All the better for us Kitty." You will see, therefore, gentlemen, that what is suggested is this: That Hall's position was such that he stood in urgent need of money, and that Cain's death would be the means of helping him to get it. That he did, fact look forward to Cain's death we shall show by remarks made by him from time to time in the presence of witnesses who will be called. For instance, we shall prove that on several different occasions he said that Cain could not possibly recover. On two occasions, when told by the men in attendance on Cain that he was better, Hall said he could not possibly get over it. On another occasion he suggested that it was a pity the doctor could not give him something to let him die easy. On the 15th January he told a man named Jackson, who had been making an invalid bed for Cain, that he was very glad he had done it so quickly, as he did not think Cain would live more than eight or nine days; and, on the afternoon of the same day, he told another witness named Stubbs that Cain was very bad indeed, and that he could not get over that night. We shall prove that on that very same day Jackson on taking the bed home was given some champagne in the sick room from a bottle which had been opened for Captain Cain, and that shortly after drinking it he became violently sick. Now, gentlemen, that the prisoner had poison in his possession of kinds which would produce symptoms such as Cain had—I mean retching, thirst, vomiting, and diarrhœa—we shall prove in this way: We shall show you that on March 20, 1885, he bought half-an-ounce of atropia eye-water; but there is some evidence that this was purchased for a foal which at the time had a weak eye. The first purchase of poison we are able to trace was on the 20th March 1885. On the 5th May 1885, we shall prove that he bought two drachms of tartar emetic, equal to about 120 grains; and we shall prove to you that from two to five grains of that drug would be sufficient to kill a man—two grains for a man in Captain Cain's state. On the 23rd May 1885 he borrowed a pestle and mortar, scales and weights (which would weigh from one grain to two drachms). and a two-ounce measure, none of which he ever returned. On the 4th November 1885 he bought another half-ounce of atropia; on the 13th November he purchased two ounces of colchicum wine; and on the 28th January 1886, the day before the captain died, he bought another half-ounce of atropia. You will see, therefore, that prisoner had plenty of poison in his possession, and it will be for you to consider what use he could have had for these poisons. So far as we know, the prisoner has given but one explanation, and that with regard to one of them only—the antimony— viz., that he used antimony for mixing with other things to make cigarettes for asthma. We shall prove that this is an unheard of use for antimony, and moreover, it is an entirely unsuitable and useless thing for the purpose. Now, gentlemen, as to the prisoner making the subject of poisons a special study. We shall prove to you that on May 9, 1885, he went to a stationer's shop in Timaru—a Mr Hutton's— and there he inquired for a book treating on antimony. Mr Hutton took down from his shelves a book called "Headland's Actions of Medicines." This book contained a chapter on the subject Hall was inquiring about, and having

7

first cut the leaves of the book at that part and glanced at them, he took the book away with him, and about a month afterwards he returned that book and then inquired for "Taylor on Poisons." Mr Hutton had a copy of this book, which prisoner borrowed. At the expiration of about a month he returned this book, borrowed it later on, and returned it again to Mr Hutton, who then suggested that he had better purchase the book, which he did, paying for it in cash at the time and making the remark "You had better not book this." These books, gentlemen, will be in evidence before you. It will be found that they contain information on the subject of antimony, colchicum, and atropia, and the extent of the knowledge prisoner was enabled to acquire from them you will be able to satisfy yourself of, if you are so minded. There is evidence of some falsification in connection with this last purchase, by the fact of the prisoner writing a date three years earlier than the date on which he bought it; also, by inserting the word "Dunedin" to indicate that he purchased it at Dunedin instead of at Timaru, as it really was; but as I am unable to explain to you what the object of this falsification can possibly be—at all events in connection with this case—I shall not remark on it. And now, gentlemen, I come to the prisoner's opportunities for administering poison. Captain Cain, as I have told you, was ill four months before his death, but only during the last five or six weeks was he subject to vomiting and other symptoms of poisoning. The exact time of his first being sick cannot be fixed with accuracy; but we shall have positive evidence that the first time his medical attendant was informed of this sickness was on December 24, 1885. As Dr Macintyre was in daily attendance on him from December 17, I shall put it to you that had the sickness been very severe or very troublesome before that the doctor would have been certain to have been informed of it. The first thing, gentlemen, as I have mentioned, that made him sick was whisky, and he could not understand how this disagreed with him, as he had been in the habit of taking it for 50 years. You will hear that it was at and after lunch that he used to vomit; that he was not sick at his breakfast or after it, but always at lunch or after lunch. You will hear, too, that at lunch he was in the habit of taking whisky, and at first it was always after the taking of the whisky that he was sick. Now we shall prove to you that there was nothing in the actual state of his health that was calculated to cause whisky to make him sick at this time; but yet, gentlemen, the fact is according to the evidence that it did so. At this time—when the sickness first began--the prisoner used to go to the house frequently, but apparently he did not go at that time for the purpose of seeing Captain Cain. The whisky which Captain Cain used was kept in a liquor-stand, containing three bottles, which stood on a cupboard in the dining room. The prisoner would have access to that stand any time that he happened to be in the dining room. We are not able to prove that at that time the prisoner carried poison about with him, but we shall be able to show that at the time of his arrest, viz., in August 1886——

Mr Chapman: Was it an arrest in connection with Cain's death?

Mr Haggitt: I did not say so. I say that we shall not be able to prove that at that time he was in the habit of carrying poisons about, although we shall be able to prove that at the time he was arrested, in August 1886, he had on his person tartar emetic in powder, and also a phial containing a solution of that poison, and that in his house was found a bottle of brandy which had been poisoned with colchicum. Now, gentlemen, as I have said that the whisky which Captain Cain used was kept on the cupboard in the dining room, it would seem to suggest a reckless disregard of consequences to say that poison was put into the whisky bottles there, as others might have taken it and suspicion would probably have been aroused; but, gentlemen, the evidence will disclose that two persons suffered from severe sickness after drinking liquor provided for the captain, and that prisoner himself provided special port wine for the men who nursed Cain at night, suggesting that it would be better to give them that rather than that they should drink the good port wine provided for the captain. Of course, gentlemen, there were other ways in which poison might have been administered than by putting it into the decanters. There may, for all we know to the contrary, have been some special glass out of which Captain Cain drank, and it might have been put into that glass; but it is suggested, at all events, that the whisky may have been poisoned for the reason that other persons were made sick by partaking of it, as some were by taking other liquors which later on were provided for Captain Cain. But though at first the prisoner did not see the captain when he called at the house, he soon afterwards became a constant visitor there. He used to call in the morning about 10 on his way to his office. He used sometimes to go in at lunch; and he used to call in again nearly every evening on his way back from his office at about 6 o'clock. During this time the captain was frequently sick. The prisoner when he went to call was left alone with Cain. If any of the household remained he requested them to leave on the plea that he had business with the captain, and he remained alone with him. The captain was frequently thirsty—one of the symptoms that would be caused by irritant poisons—and the prisoner frequently gave him drinks. Besides all these, the cough mixture and other medicines which the captain took were kept on the side table which stood just behind the bedroom door, and was hidden from the bed where the captain lay by means of a screen so that anyone lying in the bed could not see what was being done at the table where the bottles were. It will be proved to you, gentlemen, later on, that this cough mixture was a continual cause of sickness after it was administered. You will see, therefore, gentlemen, that the prisoner had plenty of opportunities for administering whatever he pleased to Captain Cain. Evidence will be given of two occasions on which the prisoner with his own hands prepared for the captain something to drink, the taking of which was immediately followed by violent sickness. One of these occasions was

8

in December, shortly before Christmas. At that time the captain was at dinner, and Mrs Ostler, Miss Gillon, Mrs Newton, and the prisoner were dining with him. The captain seemed better than usual that day, and during dinner he asked for something to drink. Hall (the prisoner) was going to give him whisky out of a decanter which stood on the table, but Cain refused it. Hall then took a glass from the table, went to the cupboard, poured some wine into a glass, put it on the table beside Cain, and poured some water into it. Shortly after drinking this Cain was seized with violent vomiting, and had to be removed from the room. On another occasion later on we shall prove that the prisoner stayed up with Captain Cain, and that on the following day Cain was continually sick. From the 1st January to the time of his death a man sat up with Cain every night—in fact, two men (Wren, a gardener, and Kay) were employed for this purpose. These men took week and week about. Kay, as I have told you, will give evidence that he noticed the cough mixture made Cain violently sick every time that he took it. We shall prove that there was nothing in the ingredients of the mixture calculated to make it act as an emetic, and we shall also prove that the chemist who mixed it up inserted nothing except what was put in the prescription. It will then be for you to consider whether anything was or might not have been added to this mixture to make it act as it did, as an emetic. We shall prove to you that Captain Cain's food did not make him sick—that he could eat jellies, custards, and things of that kind without being sick; and we shall prove that the liquor he took did not always make him feel sick. On January 13, when a bottle of champagne was opened for him by a man named Stubbs, it did not make him sick, although at other times champagne had produced sickness. We shall prove to you, moreover, that from December 19 up to the time of his death Miss Gillon gave him tea every afternoon, and that he was able to retain it without sickness following. I am forbidden in the meantime from entering into matters which I had intended commenting on to you.

His Honor : Of course you will have plenty of opportunity for commenting on the whole of the evidence.

Mr Haggitt : Yes, by-and-bye, your Honor. You will see, gentlemen, from what I have opened, what the nature of the case is, and you will see that, long as the story is, it practically resolves itself into three questions, which you will have to determine. The questions are these :—Firstly: Was antimony found in Captain Cain's body? If not, there is an end of the case, of course. Secondly: If antimony was found, did the administration of it accelerate Captain Cain's death? Thirdly: Did the prisoner administer it? These, gentlemen, are the three questions to which your attention will have to be directed. It is only with regard to the third question, gentlemen, that you can have the slightest doubt. You have heard from me the motive that it is suggested the prisoner had to wish for Captain Cain's death; you have

heard the means he had in his possession to bring that death about; you have heard the symptoms of the last illness of Captain Cain, and you have also heard the result of the analysis. The particulars of these various matters of, course, will come out in far greater detail from the evidence of the witnesses as they are examined one by one before you. The knowledge of the importance to the prisoner on the one hand and to society on the other of the conclusion at which you will have to arrive should be sufficient to secure your careful attention to the evidence that will be adduced, and I need not therefore ask it at your hands. You know your duty, gentlemen. It is simply this : that if on the evidence you are satisfied beyond a reasonable doubt that the prisoner was guilty of administering noxious drugs to Captain Cain, which acclerated his death, you are bound to find a verdict of guilty; but if, on the contrary, you have a reasonable doubt as to whether the prisoner did administer such drugs then the prisoner is entitled to the benefit of that doubt. As I have already said, gentlemen, I shall have an opportunity of commenting on the whole of the evidence after it has been given, and in the meantime I have nothing further to say to you. We shall proceed to call the witnesses.

On Mr Chapman's application all witnesses except the experts and Inspector Broham were ordered out of court.

THE EVIDENCE.

The following evidence was then taken :—

Arthur Steadman, examined by Mr White, deposed that he was manager of the Bank of New South Wales at Timaru. He knew the prisoner, who was a member of the firm of Hall and Meason, of Timaru. The firm's account was kept at the Bank of New South Wales. Hall chiefly managed and attended to the banking business. In January 1885 the firm's account on the average was overdrawn about £8000, including discount, and from that date to the 15th August the account was about the same. In December 1884 prisoner saw witness in reference to a promissory note of E. H. Cameron for £800. The note was for six months, and prisoner said that E. H. Cameron was a station manager at Waimate. The note was produced for discount and was discounted. On 13th June 1895, prisoner saw witness about another promissory note for £650, which purported to be a part renewal of the previous note. On or about 23rd September 1885 prisoner saw him about a promissory note of John Fraser's for £150 for three months. This note was also produced for discount, and was discounted. Prisoner said Fraser lived in the Mackenzie country, and gave him the document produced (memo. of transfer of mortgage) to secure the promissory note for £150. In December of 1885 prisoner saw witness respecting another promissory note—one by Mr Mitton, for £285 at three months, and said that Mitton was a station manager. These four notes were all taken away by the prisoner, the bills being renewed. Prisoner gave witness the document produced to secure Mitton's promissory note. The signature "T. Hall" in the book (poisons register) produced was in the prisoner's handwriting. Witness did not think that the prisoner's partner, Mr Meason, ever brought in any bills prior to August 1885.

Cross-examined by Mr Chapman : The liabilities to the bank amounted to about £3000. The securities held by the bank against overdraft and discounts in January 1885 were valued at £9000, and were about the same in 1886. I considered the account fairly secured. Cameron's bill for £650 was retired at due date, on the 16th of December 1885. On the 29th of January 1886 the liability to the bank was £7680. In November 1885 it was larger, being then £9800, and had been reduced in the interval. I knew Hall personally pretty well, and believe he had dogs and horses about his place. I remember on one occasion noticing something peculiar with one of Hall's eyes. It was an enlargement of the pupil of the eye. Some conversation took place about it, and Hall said he had been doing something to the eyes of one of his dogs, and thought that some of the medicine must have got into his own eye.

Re-examined : I cannot tell the date of that. Cameron's promissory note was taken up by Hall and Meason's cheque. The question of the value of the securities held had been gone into lately, and on examination the securities were found to be less than £9000, but how much less I cannot say. The securities valued in 1885 and 1886 included the promissory notes and mortgages mentioned in my evidence.

Robert Silvers Black, manager of the National Bank at Timaru, deposed : The prisoner kept his private account at our bank in January 1885, and for some time previously. In January 1885 the account was generally overdrawn something under £100. From then till the following September it ran much the same figures, increasing towards September to £200. On the 19th of November it was overdrawn £50, and from that time till the end of March the account was in credit, with one or two exceptions. In August 1886 the account was overdrawn £600, and we held security for the overdraft. The signature "T. Hall" in the book produced (the poisons register) is the prisoner's.

To Mr Denniston : We are satisfied with the security we have for the overdraft. Hall had a good commercial reputation, and might have relied upon us for £200, I think, without any special security. On December 18, 1885, Hall was in credit nearly £500, and had a substantial sum to his credit during that month, and for the whole of January.

Charles A. Wilson, a clerk, deposed : Previously to December 4, 1885, and at that time I was clerk to Hall and Meason, of Timaru. I entered their employment in 1880. I know of business transactions between Mr Cameron, a station manager at Waimate, and the firm. There were also transactions with Mr M. Mitton, station manager, Mount Peall, and with a Mr John Fraser, a shepherd in the Mackenzie country. I never received any promissory notes from any of these parties. Hall was the partner who

attended to the banking business of the firm. I may have taken promissory notes from those parties to the bank, but if I did so I received them from Hall, and took them upon his instructions. The signature in the book produced (poisons register) is Hall's. I kept the firm's ledger. In December 1884 I find an entry—" By E. H. Cameron's promissory note, December 1884, £800"; and there is a later one under "June 1885. By promissory note, 13th December, £650." Mr Mitton's account shows—"July 16, 1886. By promissory note, 19th November, £225 '; and under that the same name—"March 3, 1886. By promissory note, 15th July, £275 "; and one " January 13, 1886. By promissory note, 8th March, £205." Mr John Fraser's account shows an entry—" July 19, 1886. By promissory note, 22nd November, £150 "; and on " September 10, 1885. By promissory note, 26th December, £150." All the entries I have read are in my handwriting, and were made by Hall's instructions. Shortly after Hall's arrest there was a meeting of the creditors of the firm, and Mr W. M. Sim was appointed one of the liquidators.

This witness was not cross-examined.

Edward Hume Cameron, station manager, deposed : I know the prisoner. He belonged to the firm of Hall and Meason. I had transactions with that firm from 1881. They invested money for me. I did business with Hall personally. I got one statement showing the position of my account. (Statement produced, showing securities amounting to £1575.) Of that money I have received about £440, and have received some of the securities, purporting to be for about £500, but not worth more than from £250 to £300. There are no securities representing the balance, and I am a creditor for it. I have not received any dividend or any notice of a dividend. I gave my money to Hall personally by cheque. I never gave the firm a promissory note, nor a promissory note to anyone in my life. I have lived in that neighbourhood between 22 and 23 years. I have never heard of any other E. H. Cameron in the district.

This witness was not cross-examined.

Michael Mitton, station manager at Mount Peall, said : I know the prisoner Hall. I never gave a promissory note to the firm of Hall and Meason, or to either of the partners. I gave the firm money from time to time to invest. I chiefly gave it to the prisoner. £1480 was given in all. I have received none of the principal back, but some of the interest. I have received no dividend out of the firm's estate, and have had no intimation that any will be payable. I have lived for 26 years in South Canterbury, and never heard that there was any other person of the same name there. The signature on the transfer of mortgage produced is my name, but not my writing. I never signed any transfer of mortgage.

Cross-examined by Mr Chapman : The securities were held by the firm of Hall and Meason for me. I believe they have been since the bankruptcy handed over to someone for me.

Wilfred Wolcombe, landbroker, Timaru, and justice of the peace, said :—The document produced is a transfer of mortgage from Michael Mitton to Hall and Meason. The signature purporting to be that of the attesting witness to Mitton's signature is not mine. It is something like my writing.

John Fraser, shepherd, Mackenzie country, said :—I gave Hall and Meason money to invest for me on mortgage. I gave it to Hall—about £300 in all. I have not got the money back. It was, I believe, invested for me. I have seen one security for £150. I never gave either Hall or Meason or the firm a promissory note at any time. The signature on the transfer of mortgage produced is not mine and is nothing like it. I never signed such a transfer. They never lent me any money. It was the other way about.

William Montagu Sims, accountant and landbroker, Timaru, said :—I was appointed one of the liquidators at a meeting of the creditors of Hall and Meason, and I went carefully through the books. They showed the firm's deficiency in January 1886 to be £5207 1s 3d. In August the deficiency was £400 or £500 more than this. There is one account called Wigley's trust, of which Lysaght and Meason were trustees. There was in January £767 3s 3d due to this account by the firm of Hall and Meason. There was £928 10s 4d due to E. H. Cameron's account, and £58 8s to Mitton's account. There was also a credit to John Fraser of £277 19s.

Cross-examined by Mr Denniston : I took the debits and credits of the books, and the balance showed the deficiency. It was simply a book balance. There are plenty of land accounts, but I did not take them into consideration. I admit that if an ordinary accountant had been called in he would have made out a very different balance sheet. From information I struck out items which appeared to represent valuable assets. They represented Southland investments. Property has gone down a good deal of late.

Mr Denniston : So that a perfectly honest and straightforward firm might have been in the same position as Hall and Meason by the shrinking of values ?

Witness : It has happened in my experience. The arrest of Hall might of course have brought down the values of the assets still more. It might perhaps have altered the firm's position from a possible credit to a certain debit.

Re-examined by Mr White : All the Southland properties were left out as of no value. I took the opinion of the manager of the bank and of the clerk. I prepared what I thought wss the best statement I could get. I was acting for the creditors. There has been no particular fall in the value of property within the last year that I am aware of.

Arthur Steadman, re-called and questioned as to the Southland properties of the firm said : I had a second mortgage over 3000 acres.

Mr Chapman said this could not be proved except by the production of the document.

Witness : It proved to be a third mortgage instead of a second.

Arthur Ormsby, solicitor, Timaru, said :—I prepared a will for Mrs Hall from instructions given by herself. Previous to this the prisoner came to me. I saw Mrs Hall on 24th July 1885, and a few days before that Hall came to me. He said Mrs Hall was coming to me in a few days about a will. I prepared the will, and it was executed on 29th July 1885. It is Mrs Hall's signature on the document. I kept the will in my possession until the 4th August 1885, when I gave it to the prisoner and got his receipt for it. He called at my office expressly for it.

William Davidson, insurance agent, representing the Australian Mutual Provident Society, said :—I remember seeing the prisoner in August 1885 with reference to two life insurance proposals. He came at the beginning of the month about a proposal for a policy on his wife's life. At one of our interviews I gave him blank proposal forms. He kept them two or three days and returned them on 19th August filled up, Mrs Hall was subsequently examined by Dr Macintyre, and policies were issued by the office. They were given to Hall. I did not see Mrs Hall in connection with the policies. Hall named a stepdaughter of Captain Cain. Her name, Kate Emily Hall, appears on the policies. The luncheon adjournment here took place after which the Crown's case was resumed.

Miles Knubbley, solicitor, Timaru, said :—I knew the late Capt. Cain, and was his solicitor for six months before his death. I also knew his family. He had two stepdaughters, who were both married, one to Mr Newton and the other to the prisoner. Mrs Hall's marriage took place on May 12, 1885. Cain told me he was not on good terms with Hall. Mrs Hall kept house for him before she was married. I have known her for eight years, and during all that time she kept house for her father. Mrs Newton came backwards and forwards, but I forget who kept house after Mrs Hall's marriage. Hall and Captain Cain became friends again about November 1885. Mrs Cain died at the end of 1878. There were two settlements under which Mrs Hall became interested. The first is dated February 26, 1870. It is a settlement of certain land near Timaru. Mr Le Cren and Captain Cain became trustees of this settlement some time before his death, but at the time of his death Captain Cain, myself, and Mr Spalding were trustees under the deed. The property consisted of about 50 acres near Timaru, with the house called Woodlands upon it, where Captain Cain resided. Its capital value was about £6000 or £7000. The trust was to pay the rent of the property to Mrs Cain for her life, and after her death to her two daughters. There was an ultimate trust for the children of the latter. The net income from this property was about £480 or £500 a year. I prepared the deed of covenant to which Le Cren, Cain, Mrs Newton, and Mrs Hall were parties. It related to the same property. Its effect is to put an end to certain disputes about accounts that were pending, and also to give an annuity of £300 a year to Captain Cain and provide for the tenancy of the house. The deed is executed by all the parties. The other settlement refers to two lots in Timaru, which Captain Cain settled on his wife and two stepdaughters. The trust is now vested in Mr Spalding and myself. The net value of this property was about £2000. It produced a little over £200 a year. The trust was to apply the income to pay off the mortgage on the property, and then to apply it for the benefit of Mrs Cain, his stepdaughters, and their children. Cain had other property besides that included in this trust. I am one of the executors under his will. The will is dated 22nd December 1885, and there is a codicil dated 6th January 1886. Certain legacies are bequeathed, and the real estate of the testator goes to his wife and stepdaughters, and the residue to a nephew who was in New Zealand a short time ago. A little under £3000 was left altogether. I produce a settlement made by Mrs Hall in 1881 before her marriage. It purports to deal with nine acres of land exactly opposite Woodlands. There are really only seven acres, and it is approximately worth about £200 an acre. There is an endorsement dated March 1886 which gives the power to deal with the property by deed during her life. Mrs Hall was also entitled to about £2000 in money in addition to the £1400, the value of this land. There is also a will of Mrs Cain, for which letters of administration were granted. Mrs Newton and Mrs Hall were the beneficiaries under the will. The value of the entire property was about £500 between them. The prisoner made inquiries of me about the trust properties several times since January 1886. He wanted to know how they stood and what he might expect from it. I gave him later on the information he required. I made out an account of the trust properties and gave it to him in July 1886.

Cross-examined by Mr Denniston: Captain Cain's estate, which I value at £3000, consisted of shares mostly. There was a debt to the Bank of New South Wales, to which Cain had guaranteed Newton's overdraft. I cannot say of my own knowledge that Hall knew anything of Cain's position. Till the deed of covenant on December 5, two months before Cain's death, the position of Mrs Hall and Mrs Newton would not have been altered legally by his death. I acted in the preparation of this deed. It was a perfectly voluntary deed as far as Mrs Hall was concerned. She lost by the deed, practically surrendering some claim she might have had against the trust estate and getting nothing. Hall was aware of the execution of this deed and its terms. Mrs Hall used to be guided by his wishes in her business, but as to this particular deed he left her to do as she thought proper. He was consulted by her about it, and made appointments for her to have it executed. That was the first deed that gave Captain Cain an interest in the trust property, Woodlands, and it was executed by Mrs Hall with Hall's consent. There was a friendly suit to rectify the position of the parties. Captain Cain swore an affidavit in this suit about a fortnight before he died. He assented to the suit. I explained the nature of the affidavit and the proceedings to him. I ex-

plained that the affidavit was for the purpose of assisting the suit. As far as I know, he had very friendly feelings towards Hall at this time. I saw him on 28th January, and he was still concurrent in the matter. All the property left to Mrs Hall and Mrs Newton consisted of some household furniture and some land, worth about £140, near Timaru. It is bringing in nothing at present. Most of the furniture was sold and Hall bought a large portion of it. Hall was living in a house with 10 acres of land, worth about £50 a year. One result of Captain Cain's death was his moving into the larger place Woodlands, and some consequent expenditure. Nothing that Hall ever said to me showed any knowledge of the contents of Cain's will. On my last visit to Cain he was very feeble. I cannot say he was cheerful. At other times during his illness he was sometimes cheerful. He was a man who always enjoyed a joke.

Re-examined by Mr Haggitt: The furniture I spoke of was taken by Hall as Mrs Hall's share. I have heard since that Hall was looking for a house before Captain Cain's death. When he moved into Woodlands he was to pay me £83 a year rent. The last half-year's rent has been paid by Mrs Hall since the prisoner has been in gaol.

Frederick Le Cren (manager for the N.Z.L. and M.A. Company at Timaru) deposed : I knew Captain Cain very well, having been acquainted with him for 30 years. He had lived at Timaru for 20 years, and was an old merchant captain. His wife died in 1878, leaving Captain Cain with two stepdaughters, Kate Emily Espie and Jane Espie. I was a trustee with Captain Cain of some property which had been bought in the name of Kate Emily Espie. Miss Espie made this over to her stepfather a long time before her marriage. Captain Cain did not approve of his stepdaughter's marriage with the prisoner. He was in Dunedin when the marriage took place, and was not on good terms with Hall at the time. He was in Dunedin expressly to get away from being present at the marriage. I knew the prisoner personally, and had conversations with him with respect to the trust I held for his wife. The first conversation was before the marriage, and had reference to the trust that Miss Kate Emily Espie had made of her own property. I met him in the street and told him I had written to Miss Espie, hearing that she was to be married, and recommended her to appoint another trustee. He replied, "Oh, I have seen Kitty, and have decided to let it remain as it is, and not release you. The deed is all right." My reply was that I should prefer to be out of it. In the month of August I was in his office and he was asking me about these trust moneys. I told him her father had the management of it, and he would be able to get all particulars, no doubt, from him. He replied, " I don't know about that; you will have to be responsible as well." I said, " Very well; but I think it would be better, considering the feelings that exist, to let things go on as they are while the old man lives." I then left him, and afterwards told Cain the nature of the conversations. I saw the prisoner again, I think in December, and told him Captain Cain objected to my resigning the trust. At that time he suggested that the deed might be cancelled as it has not been stamped. To that I objected. Later on he said he had a way out of the difficulty by a friendly action, and that I need not defend it. I was served with a writ on the 26th or 27th of January, and the action went by default. About April I paid the money over to him—about £750. I did nothing at all in the action. I paid the money to Hall personally, on an order from Mrs Hall, but I think there was also an order from the court. No one acted for me in that action. Hall used to ask me what moneys I had in hand, and what I was doing with them. That was in the latter part of 1885. I told him that any money I had in hand I would deposit in the bank. To that he was quite agreeable. He asked me what I had in hand, and I told him. The deed of release produced is what I called Mrs Hall's receipt. I saw an order of the court to give it up, and I obtained this deed of release. I remember an interview with Hall in the middle of December, and told him then that Captain Cain wished me to remain with him in the trust, and that as long as he (Captain Cain) lived he would not give up the trust. I used frequently to visit Captain Cain, and saw him up to within three days of his death. I do not think he came to Timaru much after the New Year, and do not recollect seeing him in town after Christmas. He used to drive down at about 10 o'clock, walk about town and be driven back to lunch. Captain Cain was about 70 years of age, but he was able to get out of his carriage and look after any little business he had to attend to. During December I saw him two or three times a week. We used to play whist together at his house up to about the end of November. Up to that time he was in fairly good health, but his sight was failing him. So far as I know, he used to drink whisky up to the end of November. He drank nothing but whisky, and up to that time I never heard him complain that it did not agree with him. Some time in December, so far as I recollect, he had to give up whisky, and he remarked that it was an extraordinary thing the whisky used to make him sick. This was about the beginning of December, for he asked me to get him a turkey for Christmas. I did not see him take whisky for two months before he died, but I saw him violently sick the Sunday before Christmas Day. He told me he had been recommended to take rum, and that he could not make it out, but he was sick after taking that. The whisky Captain Cain drank was specially imported by my brother. I took the same class of whisky, but it never made me sick. I did not drink whisky in Captain Cain's house after the beginning of November, if I took it so late as that time. That was the only time I saw Captain Cain sick. Miss Gillon was staying at Captain Cain's in January, and I think I remember being there once when she brought in tea, and I had some. I cannot say whether Captain Cain had any. I never found Captain Cain alone after Christmas ; there was generally some friend with him. Denis Wren and Kay were with him at different times, and at other times Mrs Newton or

Miss Gillon was present. In January Captain Cain was removed to the dining room, his bed being placed there. A table stood in the corner of the room, the bedstead was behind the door, and there was a French window in front of him, at the foot of the bed, and a screen between the door and the bed. From the time Captain Cain got the bed in the dining room he never rose from it to my knowledge. I do not think that Captain Cain and Hall became friendly until the latter part of October, or probably later.

Cross-examined by Mr Denniston : At first I was a trustee in all the trusts, and my duties so far as the children were concerned commenced on the death of Mrs Cain. I did not study the trust deeds very carefully, but I knew the terms of the trust generally. There was no appointment of guardian in relation to these trusts. I took no part in the trusts, and was a mere name in connection with them. Captain Cain told me everything was kept right, and I relied upon that, knowing him so long and his relationship to the daughters. I acquiesced in the suit instituted by Hall on Mrs Hall's behalf. Captain Cain was an abstemious man ; I never knew him to take more than two glasses in an evening, and he took it very weak. I do not remember his complaining that champagne made him sick. I am reported to have said that Captain Cain complained that he was sick after taking his whisky and after taking his meals. He also told me that he took whisky at his lunch. The table in the dining room is visible in daylight from the verandah.

Re-examined : I do not know where the whisky was kept after the dining room was used as a bedroom. Previously it was kept on the cupboard in that room. I saw medicine bottles on the table behind the door.

Dr Hogg, medical practitioner, of Timaru, said :—I know Bridget Wren, wife of Denis Wren. I saw her on Thursday, the morning before I started. She was ill at her house at Timaru—about to be confined—and was not in a fit state to travel; she would not be under a fortnight or three weeks.

The depositions of Bridget Wren were then read in substance as follows :—I am the wife of Denis Wren, gardener, of Timaru. I was domestic servant to the late Captain Cain up to the time of his death. He was ill about four months before he died. He was ill about 18 months before that, and during this illness he lost the small toe of the right foot. The captain was very sick at times, and first began to vomit about four months before his death. The captain was not very bad about this time. Mr and Mrs Newton were at the house shortly before he commenced to vomit. Mrs Hall used to come to the house. Mr Hall came sometimes, but did not see the captain. Mr Paterson stopped at the house one week at about the time the captain became sick. I cannot remember if the captain vomited before or after Paterson came. The captain was sick before Hall made up friends with him. I cannot remember the month the captain commenced to vomit. He was taken to his bed. He commenced to vomit two months before taking to his bed. On the 1st December last Mrs Newton and Miss Houston came, and

Miss Gillon came afterwards, as also myself and Denis Wren. We were not married then. Newton did not come occasionally to the house in December. Hall first commenced to call and see Cain about three months before he died. He used to come in the morning about 10 o'clock nearly every morning, and sometimes at luncheon time. I only remember him coming about twice to luncheon. The captain had lunch at the same table on one of these occasions. Hall used also to call at the house on his way home from the office about 6 o'clock. He used to call in nearly every evening and remain half an hour—sometimes less. Only twice, so far as I can remember, did Hall come back and sit with the captain, The nights followed one another, and were before Christmas—the one being the night before and the other Christmas Eve. I saw Mrs Newton in the dining room at 11 o'clock. I heard her say she was going to sit up with the captain also, and believed from this she did sit up. After Christmas George Kay came and used to attend on the captain. I think I did see the captain vomit before November, but how long before I cannot remember. In December he was oftener sick than in November He used to vomit in the middle of and after lunch—not every time, but pretty often. The captain used to take whisky with his lunch, and he used to vomit after taking it. I am quite sure it was at luncheon time that he was sick, not before or after breakfast. Mr Paterson, as well as I can remember, left the house about three months before the captain's death. Mrs Newton left about the same time; it might have been a few days later.

Cross-examination: In his first illness he vomited one day; that is all I can remember. The captain got better after a few days, and was able to get up. As far as I know the illness lasted only a few days. He was in bed only a few days. He was a good while bad with his foot. The whisky that Captain Cain used was in the sick room in a liquor stand with three bottles. The three all contained whisky. I do not remember the liquor stand being taken out of the room. If any person wanted whisky they could take it from the spirit stand. If any person came to the house they would get it from the stand in the sick room. I noticed one of the captain's hands very much swollen on his last illness. I do not know whether Hall saw Captain Cain every time he called. He could have seen him unknown to me. I have seen champagne in the sick room. It had a tap bored through the cork; the corks were not drawn.

By the Court: He went to bed in consequence of his vomiting during his first illness. There was more whisky in a jar in the storeroom. I do not know of whisky being anywhere else in the house except in the sick room. The dining room was turned into the sick room for about four weeks before he died. The spirits were kept on a sideboard at this time. There were no spirits in the cupboard.

Dr Martin, practising in Dunedin, said: I am attending Jane Ellis Newton, a witness in this case. She was confined on the 17th inst., and could not attend the court for about a fortnight.

The depositions of Mrs Newton were then, read in substance as follows:—I reside at Melbourne. The accused married my sister in May of 1885. Shortly after the marriage I went to reside at Woodlands, the residence of the late Captain Cain, and, with the exception of occasional absences, remained there till his death. At the time of the marriage my father and the accused were not on good terms; they afterwards got on good terms and became friendly. Hall, I think, first began to visit Woodlands on friendly terms about the beginning of November. I was twice away from the house on a visit between June and the beginning of January. Between November and January I was not absent, but I was away about the beginning of November. From the end of November to the end of January Hall was a frequent visitor to the house. On my return to the house in the beginning of November Hall called to see me. It was the end of November before he began to see the captain. He used to pay his first visits to the captain in the mornings. He used to call every morning, and that continued up to the time of Cain's death. He would stay 10 minutes or so with the captain during these calls. I think there were no other persons present besides Hall and the captain at any of these interviews. Hall used to call again after office hours frequently through the week. He used to see the captain at those calls. There was a nurse with Cain. I think he always left the room when visitors came. Towards the last Hall called once or twice at 10 o'clock at night. On two occasions he sat up with the captain all night. This was about Christmas time; but whether they were consecutive nights or at different times I don't know. I was in the captain's room several times when Hall entered. Hall used to speak to me. He used to say, "I have business; I want to speak to your father." He made no other request to me that I remember. I used to leave the room in consequence of what Hall said to me. Hall on coming in would say, "How are you this morning, captain?" I have heard him also ask the captain if he had had anything lately. The captain always wanted something to drink, as he was suffering from thirst. I have seen Hall give the captain champagne and his cough mixture. The captain used to ask for the latter from all his visitors. I cannot say if I ever saw Hall give him anything else, but I don't think I did. Whisky and port wine were kept in the room also. The captain used to take port wine, I think, not whisky at this time. The things I have mentioned were kept on a table in the sick room from the time the captain took to his bed. These things were kept on a table and in a cupboard behind a screen in the dining room. I cannot say when the captain first began to vomit. It was an "old thing" so far as I know. I saw father sick soon after I returned to the house in November, but don't remember if he made any remark. I do not know what he attributed his sickness to. He was sometimes sick before lunch. He was in the habit of taking a glass of wine or whisky the first part of his illness. He would take either a glass of wine, whisky, or rum when,

14

he returned from his drive. He gave as a reason for giving up drinking whisky that it made him sick. He said it was a strange thing that after drinking whisky for 20 years it should now make him sick. After this he took brandy, but not liking it he took port wine, taking the port wine to the end. I remember dining one day with Mr Ostler, Miss Gillon, Hall, and my father, and the latter asking for something to drink. I think it was the first time Hall had been to lunch. I remember the captain asking for something to drink. Hall was going to get the whisky from a decanter on the table when the captain said, "Not whisky; it makes me sick." Someone then said to Hall, "The wine is in the cupboard." Hall then took a glass from the table and went to the cupboard and poured out some wine. It was port or sherry. I do not know which for certain. I believe it was port. He put the glass on the table, but I did not notice the contents particularly. Hall next poured some water into the glass and put it alongside of the captain. I did not remain long in the room after this, as I was ill and went out. I could not see what Hall poured out at the cupboard, as his back was to me. I could not say if he was standing up or stooping. I took no particular notice of him. The captain was blind of one eye. At this time there were two bottles of whisky in the sick room, both in the same liquor stand. There were no bottles of whisky in the other rooms. There was none in any other decanter or bottle in the house. There was no whisky in a special decanter for visitors.

Cross-examined: From the time I came back in November up to the time Hall became friendly I saw the captain sick. Hall did not see my father then that I know of.

By the Court: I said, in answer to Mr Perry's question, that I was told he was sick. It was after I came back from Dunedin that my father and Hall were reconciled. I heard before I returned that they had spoken. I cannot say whether I was present when they were reconciled, or whether the reconciliation took place days or weeks after I returned from Dunedin. I do not remember whether I heard from Hall that there was an interview between himself and my father before I returned. I do not think my sister told me in Hall's presence that there had been an interview or reconciliation during my absence. I made a mistake. I returned to Woodlands from Dunedin about two days before the Timaru show, and it was a few days after that I saw my father vomit once. I can only say once safely. This was at lunch. I think there was only myself present. He was very sick, and it was the only time I saw him sick about this period.

Jowsey Jackson, blacksmith, Timaru, said:— On the 11th or 12th of January last I received an order from the prisoner to make an invalid bedstead. He saw me and said the bed was to be ready as soon as possible. On the 15th he saw me again and said he was glad I had got on with it so well; he did not think Captain Cain would live any longer than eight or nine days. The same day I took the bed to Woodlands and helped to place the captain on it. We brought him out of the room he had been occupying into the larger room. George Kay gave me a little champagne, which he got from the bedroom from which the captain had been brought. The bottle had a patent stopper with a tap in it. The cork had not been drawn, but the tap had been passed through it. About an hour after drinking the champagne I felt very sick, but did not vomit. I was bad from about half-past 12 to 6 or 7 in the evening. I never before felt sick in that way. I had taken nothing that morning before the champagne, except my breakfast. I never had a sick attack like this before.

Cross-examined by Mr Chapman: This was about half-past 12 or 1 o'clock. I generally breakfast at about 8. I was sitting in the room into which Cain was brought. He walked in with the assistance of Kay and Denis Wren. I went into the small room he had occupied afterwards, and Kay reached down the champagne and gave me some. The syphon was in it then. The wine was not fizzing much. I think the shank of the syphon went pretty nearly down to the bottom of the bottle, which was about three-parts full.

George William Gardiner, residing at Timaru, said: I owned a house at Timaru last year, and hearing some time in January last year that Hall wanted one, I went to him and offered to let him mine as I was going to take a voyage to England. He said, "I have been inquiring for a house, but to tell you the real truth I don't want to get one because the old man will be dead in a day or two, and we will be getting his house." Captain Cain died about a fortnight after that conversation. He used to be one of my employers, and when Hall had this conversation with me I said "Is it too late to visit him?" and Hall said he supposed it was.

Cross-examined by Mr Chapman: I believe I have just repeated the exact words, as far as my memory serves me. I could not pledge myself to them. I do not think the words were that Captain Cain might die any day. I think the words were that he expected the old man would be dead in a day or two. He made no mention of the doctor. I can swear positively he did not. I only knew that the captain was unwell, and was surprised to hear of his being so ill. He was one of the directors of the Timaru Herald Company, with which I was employed. He always came to the office once a month.

At this stage the court adjourned until the following morning at 10 o'clock.

TUESDAY, JANUARY 25.

Thomas Hall was again placed in the dock upon the charge that he, on the 9th of January 1886, did feloniously, wilfully, and with malice aforethought, kill and murder one Henry Cain. Mr B. C. Haggitt (Crown prosecutor at Dunedin), assisted by Mr White (Crown prosecutor at Timaru), appeared for the Crown; Mr F. R. Chapman, with him Mr J. E. Denniston (instructed by Mr Perry, of Timaru) for the defence.

The hearing of this case was resumed at 10 o'clock.

Denis Wren (examined by Mr White) deposed: I am a gardener, and was formerly in the employment of Captain Cain. I was with him for two years before he died and up to the time of his death. Eighteen months before he died he suffered from a severe illness, and lost the little toe of the right foot. The prisoner began visiting the house three or four months before the death of Captain Cain. When he first visited the house he might have seen Captain Cain, but he did not speak to him. Prisoner began seeing Captain Cain on friendly terms three or four months before the captain's death, and he then called more frequently than before. He called three times a day some part of the time the captain was ill, but mostly twice. His first visit would be about 10 o'clock or a little after, and he would remain with the captain about 10 minutes. The next visit would be paid in the evening at about 6 o'clock, and sometimes, but not often, he would call at about 1 o'clock. The morning and evening visits were made daily. At those visits prisoner used to see the captain alone. When he came in the evening he would remain half an hour or an hour, and sometimes till 10 o'clock. I have known him to call later than 7 or 8 o'clock. Twice, I think, he remained with the captain all night. Those occasions were, I think, about the 23rd and 24th of December 1885. I have been in the sick room when Hall has called. I was first employed in nursing Captain Cain about Christmas. Kay and myself were appointed to look after the captain. From Christmas to the time of his death I was a great deal with the captain. Someone was with him day and night. I used sometimes to remain in the sick room when Hall called, but he requested me to leave on a few occasions, saying he wanted to speak to the captain in private. Sometimes I would go out, but oftener I would remain in, if I was engaged doing anything for the captain. After I had done what I was doing for the captain when Hall entered, I would not remain in the room, but would leave them together. I remember being sent a day or two before Christmas Day by the captain for Hall. Captain Cain first became sick, I think, some time before Christmas, in December. That was the first time I saw him sick, so far as I can remember. I do not know what he had taken then, or if he had taken anything. During his illness the captain remarked to me that he could not understand how it was the whisky made him sick; that he had been used to it all his lifetime, and it had never made him sick before. That remark was only made once, so far as I can remember. After Christmas Hall said to me that the captain could not possibly get better. The captain took to his bed for good about 12 or 13 days before his death. He was at that time moved into another room. There was a table in the sick room, on which was kept medicine, champagne for the captain, and whisky. The whisky was kept in a spirit stand, and there were tumblers on the table. There were several kinds of medicine. The captain was not able to help himself from the table, but was assisted by whoever was in the room. I saw the captain every night. The night before

his death I went into the bedroom at about 11 o'clock before going to bed, as it was not my night to sit up. I thought the captain looked very well that night, and he was in very good spirits. His voice sounded very fair for a man in his condition. He said, "Have not you gone to bed, Jimmy?" I said, "No; I have come to bid you good night, captain." He said, "It's time you went to bed," and I then left him. I had no special wine or spirits provided for me at first, but when the captain knocked off drinking whisky Mrs Newton provided whisky for me. It was about the same time that the invalid bedstead was brought home that Mrs Newton provided whisky for me. I first began sitting up with the captain at Christmas time, and I would then sometimes take wine or spirits through the night. I took the wine or spirits from the bottles in the sick room, and afterwards from the dining room. There was no whisky in the stand when the bottle was provided for me, and the whisky stand was then in the sideboard. I went on one occasion to where Hall lived by the direction of Cain. That was on the 23rd of December. I told him that Cain was not very well, and he remarked he was glad he'd made friends with the old chap. I could not say whether the medicines disagreed with Cain. He was so often sick I could not say what made him sick. He first kept to the house in the middle of December, and did not go to town after that time. Previously he used to go to town daily, being driven down in a buggy at about 10 o'clock, and remaining there till 1 o'clock, when he would be driven back. I was generally with him on those occasions. He was not sick on his way to and from town. I used to see him after his lunch at that time, as he would then come out on the verandah and smoke his pipe. I do not remember seeing Captain Cain smoke after he took to his bed. Cross-examined by Mr Chapman: After Christmas I have seen him smoking in his bed, and after I began to sit up with him. It takes about 10 minutes to drive from Woodlands to Timaru. I was groom and gardener and had various duties to perform outside the house, but nothing specially to do inside the house until I had to take care of the captain. Hall used to come always to Woodlands so far as I know, but at first he would only see Mrs Newton or leave Mrs Hall and call for her again. I have seen the captain pass Hall by in the street and not speak to him. What I observed before I entered the house as nurse was that Captain Cain and Hall were not on speaking terms. When I entered the house I had better opportunities of seeing what took place between the captain and Hall. Hall came on two occasions to sit up all night, and I saw him at 12 o'clock one night, as he called me up to help the captain. After that hour I cannot say what became of Hall. The captain was sick nearly every day from the time I went into the house. I heard of his being sick before, but do not know how long before I did not hear of his vomiting during his former illness. I heard of his being sick at lunch, but I could not say how long that was before I went to act as nurse. Captain Cain was coughing a good deal when I went into the house, and he complained of the pain round his back and in his chest. When he coughed it used to make him sick. The coughing did not always make him sick, but if he took anything to drink directly after it used to make him sick. He used to suffer a good deal from thirst. I gave him champagne, and whisky 'and water, and brandy and water. I used sometimes to draw the champagne. We drew it with a champagne tap. The tap had a bent nozzle, and the shank reached nearly to the bottom of the bottle. The screen projected about half a foot behind the end of the bed so as to keep off the draught. I sometimes had conversations with Hall as to how the captain was. I did not think the captain was in a dangerous state, but thought he would get over it. The doctor said he was dropsical, and a waterproof sheeting was put under his legs. Captain Cain had other visitors besides Hall, and sometimes I stayed in the room and sometimes I left. I was glad to get the chance of leaving, and I could leave if they were intimate friends. I do not rember any conversation with the captain about his dying. Captain Cain used to talk a good deal to me, and would sometimes make jokes. When the captain ceased to use whisky the stand was left in the same place, on the top of the cupboard. Sometimes there was whisky in the bottles, but I do not remember there being any put in the bottles in the stand after the captain was taken to the large room. The captain was not so sick during the latter end of his illness as he was at the commencement of it.

Re-examined by Mr Haggitt: I commenced to nurse the captain about Christmas time. I think I sat up with the captain a night before Hall sat up with him. I last drove the captain out about the middle of December, and before that time had not sat up with him. I do not remember the captain smoking after he was moved to the dining room. Kay made the captain smoke, and the captain used to get us to smoke to sweeten the room. I did not see the captain smoke in his regular way until after Christmas. I used to leave the captain at Le Cren's office, and then call for him. This was a daily matter, and I do not remember seeing him sick at any time I was out with him. I remember seeing the captain pass Hall in the street; that was three or four months before Cain's death. Although not on speaking terms, Hall used to call at the house. Sometimes he would go in and sometimes he would not. He would generally go into the house when he called in the evening. I think Hall called me up on both nights that he stayed with the captain. The captain had not been sick when he called me. I was there the next day after the prisoner had been sitting up with the captain. Miss Gillon was there, and I remember the captain was very sick that day—Christmas Day. I do not remember what he was taking then. I do not think he was taking cough mixture, and do not remember if he was taking any medicine. At that time he was taking his whisky, and I believe he took whisky that day. I do not remember, but I might have given him some myself. I used to give him things at night—tea and biscuit. The tea did not make him sick. I used to make the tea in the kit-

chen. He took the tea right to the end without being sick. I used also to give him custards and jellies. He took them to the end, and they did not make him sick that I remember. I was attending Captain Cain all day on the day before he died. Miss Gillon used to come and see him. I do not remember her giving him anything that afternoon. I think Captain Cain had some chicken the day before he died, and that he ate some of it; but I do not remember anything specially about it. He appeared to me better that day, and I was surprised next morning when I heard he was dying. He was less sick I think on that day. I was giving him some brandy and water and his medicine at that time. When I left at 8 o'clock Kay and Mr Stubbs succeeded me. I went in about 11 o'clock, and he then appeared all right—rather better than usual. The next thing that happened was my being called at 5 o'clock in the morning. He was speechless and dying then, but he did not die for five hours. He could speak till 2 o'clock. I was with him from 5 in the morning till a few minutes before he died. His complexion was altered, and I observed the swelling had gone down from his hands and feet. He was speechless after 5 o'clock, but was breathing freely. There was no doctor present after 5 o'clock. He was then breathing heavily with a rumbling noise in his throat. His ordinary complexion was reddish, but it changed on the day he died. Once or twice after he was moved into the big room he appeared to see things, and called out that someone was coming. This was not sudden waking out of sleep. He never used to sleep much. This happened two or three times. He had an attack of severe diarrhœa after Christmas, which continued during his illness. I don't remember that he got excited at any time, nor low spirited. He continued to be fond of a joke down to the last. The champagne tap produced is like the one that was used. [The tap produced had a long thin tube which would reach to the bottom of the bottle.] I used to put it about half-way down at first, and as the champagne got lower the tube was pressed down. The cork had to be drawn for the last of the bottle. The champagne was generally given by whoever was in the room. The captain took two quart bottles of champagne in the morning and sometimes two more bottles at night.

Mr Haggitt: A very good allowance, your Honor.

Mr Denniston: Yes; and yet he complained of getting sick!

Witness: He used to take a little champagne always. At the time he took the four bottles a day he took no food. Just at the last he took brandy and some food again, his champagne being limited. I never saw the prisoner giving Cain champagne. The thirst continued down to the last. When I said he was better Hall once remarked to me that he thought he could never get over it. It was only for about a day that the captain took port wine. I drank port wine when I was sitting up and sometimes champagne, but very seldom. I took champagne out of a newly-opened bottle or out of a bottle which I opened myself, as the circumstances required. The cough medicine stood on a table inside the door. The cough mixture was in ordinary medicine bottles which would hold about three or four wineglassfuls. I don't know when he first began to take the cough mixture. He did not take any before Christmas, but he took it down to the last. I gave him some on January 28. A bottle of the mixture would last a day or half a day. There were two bottles, and we had to mix the dose. He took it when he coughed. It was an effervescent mixture.

To his Honor: I used to fetch the medicine sometimes from the chemist (Watkin's), but sometimes it was sent up. I have no reason to believe any medicine excepting that prescribed by the doctor was taken. I administered the medicine in accordance with the doctor's instructions.

To Mr Chapman: There might be a dozen bottles on the table. I could not say that the captain was taking champagne when Hall sat up. He always took it. When I took anything it was generally at night when I was sitting up. I took champagne at odd times, but not often. I did not drink brandy or port wine. On the last occasion I gave the captain brandy he only moistened his lips. The reason the wine was stopped was because it made him sick. Mrs Newton was the housekeeper, and looked after the supplies. She saw that we had what we wanted.

Margaret Graham Houston (examined by Mr Haggitt) said: I knew the late Captain Cain. I went to his house on the 1st of December. I had met him twice before at Woodlands. I had never stayed in the house before this time. Mrs Newton was a friend of mine, and I knew Mrs Hall too. When I first went there only Mrs Newton, Captain Cain, and myself were the residents. Denis Wren and Bridget, now Mrs Wren, were the servants. Mrs Newton's little boys were also there. There were two of them, aged five and nine years. Miss Gillon came to live there just before Christmas. George Kay came afterwards to nurse Captain Cain. When I first went Captain Cain was in fairly good health. He was taken ill about a week before Christmas. The first that I knew of his illness was after he had met Dr Macintyre, and he had been told that he had dropsy. He was not altogether well before that time, but he was getting about as usual. We all had our meals together till the captain was ill. It was after Christmas that he had to be laid up, and then he took his meals away from us. I have known him to go out of the room from meals saying he felt sick. This occurred once or twice—once at tea and once at lunch. It was after he told me he had seen Dr Macintyre. He used to take water and wine at his meals — sometimes port and sometimes sherry. He didn't take whisky during any of the time I was there. I saw him sick once after the time he did not come to meals. I had not seen him sick up till Christmas, but I had heard about it from Captain Cain and Bridget. I think it was the beginning of January when I first saw him sick. I think George Kay was attending to him then. I was attending to him for a fortnight before Kay

came. He then went on getting worse. Wren attended to him at nights occasionally about a week before Kay came. Sometimes he sent him away.

Witness spoke in a very low tone of voice during this examination and had to be repeatedly told to speak louder. Eventually the witness began to cry, and——

Mr Haggitt said if she did not feel well he would take another witness.

Miss Houston then at once left the witness-box and retired to the witnesses' room.

Florence Gillon, a governess by occupation, living at Wellington, deposed: I knew the late Captain Cain, also Mrs Newton and Mrs Hall. On the 19th December 1885 I went on a visit to Woodlands. I had very often been there before. I went there in December on a Saturday from Dunedin. Captain Cain was ill and had been ill for some time before I went there, but he was up when I arrived. Mrs Newton, Miss Houston, Captain Cain, Denis, and Bridget were in the house at that time. On the Monday evening I was in the room with Captain Cain. He said he felt ill and would have to go to bed. I assisted him to his bedroom and called Denis. His room was next to the dining room, where we were. I could not tell the nature of his illness. This was after tea, about 6 or 7. He did not get up the next morning. I saw him the next day in his room. I could not say whether he got up on Wednesday. My impression is that he did not leave his room on that day. I went to see him every day and read the morning paper to him. Sometimes in the afternoon I used to read a book to him. I used to be with him about half-an-hour—perhaps more. He was very ill on Thursday and did not get up. On Thursday night I went out to where the prisoner used to live, about four miles from Woodlands. I stayed all night there. Hall stayed all night at Woodlands so that I should stay with his wife at their house. About 10 next morning, Christmas Day, I returned to Woodlands. The boy drove Mrs Hall and me over. I have no distinct recollection of seeing Captain Cain that morning, but I was told he was very ill. I went to church, and then came back to Woodlands. I think Bridget and Denis were out when I came back. I sat with Captain Cain that afternoon for two or three hours. He was sick and vomiting nearly the whole afternoon. I don't remember having seen him sick before that day. The doctor came that afternoon. He was not sent for. It was about 4 o'clock when he came. After he left Bridget came, and Mrs Newton and Miss Houston were also in attendance. I saw Hall at Woodlands on the 19th. On the afternoon of Christmas Day I gave Captain Cain his medicine for his cough, and champagne. That was all I had ever given him. The medicine did not make him any better. The sickness still continued. When I found the cough medicine did not do any good I stopped giving it to him. I gave him champagne all the time. The champagne was standing there. There was a patent tap like the one produced in the bottle. I always saw the tap in the bottles after that. I had never seen it in the house before. I told the doctor what I had done. After the doctor left I don't remember going in to stay with Captain Cain. All the time I was at Woodlands I read to him if he was not ill. I remember he was a little better after Christmas Day. I got up at 4 o'clock on New Year's morning to relieve someone else who had been sitting up. I left him at 7 o'clock. The servant was up then. He talked sometimes while I was sitting with him. I brought him some tea at 7 o'clock. He was not sick after it. I often took him tea in the afternoon about half-past 2. I made the tea myself in the kitchen, and generally took some myself. He always took the tea, and I never heard of it having made him sick. It was later on that I read to him. He seemed to like the tea. George Kay came on New Year's Day, and I had no more nursing to do after that. Captain Cain told me he had not enough to eat and that he had not been properly fed. At another time he said he had had too much to eat and that it had made him sick. He used to speak to me about Mr Hall. I recollect the 28th January, the day before he died. I sat with him that evening about 7 o'clock, and gave him some chicken, which he ate and seemed to like. He took a dinnerplate full. I did not hear of his being sick after that. I had no fear for him at that time. Miss Houston was still living in the house on that occasion. I know that someone was invited to the house that evening by Mrs Newton.

Mr Denniston raised some objection to this evidence.

His Honor said he supposed it was to show that Cain was not very bad.

Mr Haggitt said that was the object.

His Honor: I'm not sure that it could be taken strictly as evidence if it were objected to.

Mr Haggitt: Very well, we'll leave it.

Witness: I remember on one occasion driving with Hall to his place when he referred to Captain Cain. He said it was a pity the doctors did not give him something to help him to die, he seemed to be struggling so much. I remember meeting Mr and Mrs Hall at the door of Woodlands one day during the earlier part of my visit there. They were coming out of their dogcart. I said Captain Cain had just been making another will. Mr Hall said, "All the better for us, Kitty." He appeared pleased. I have heard the prisoner saying that Captain Cain was not likely to recover. I think I heard him say so on more than one occasion. I remember on one occasion providing for the men who sat up with the captain. I was given a bottle of whisky by Mrs Newton to take into the sick room for the men. This was not long before Captain Cain's death. I left it in the bottle. I had no reason to think it was decanted. The prisoner told me he had provided inferior port wine for the men so that the good would not go so quickly. Hall came frequently to the house in the morning on his way to the office, and in the evening on his way home. I remember once his coming to lunch.

Mr Haggitt at this stage intimated that he had still a number of questions to ask, and as it was half-past 1 o'clock the usual adjournment for luncheon was made.

After the luncheon adjournment, Mr Chapman resumed the cross-examination of Mrs Gillon.

Witness: Hall was at the house more frequently than his wife, but he sometimes brought her in the morning and left her, and called for her again in the evening. He always came to the verandah and called at any rate, but did not always stop any time. While I was there Mrs Newton was the housekeeper, and when I went for something once, it was from her I got the keys. I heard from Hall afterwards of the special wine being provided for the men to drink. I heard of no restriction being put upon the two men as to what they might take until I gave out the one bottle to them. There was nothing to prevent me, if I had chosen, taking champagne from the bottle in use. Hall's remark about the captain which I mentioned before was that it was a pity they did not give him something, he was suffering so much. Captain Cain suffered from his cough and from weariness and inability to move about. I never was before in a house where people were in a dying state, and do not remember hearing such a remark made before. Captain Cain's condition was discussed sometimes in the house—as to whether he would get over it, and how long he would last.

Miss Houston was then recalled.

Mr Haggitt suggested that the best thing would be for someone—Mr Denniston, if he liked—to stand by the witness and repeat her answers, as they were inaudible to the court.

His Honor thought the examining counsel would be the best person to do that.

Mr Haggitt: I am quite willing, only I do not wish it to be said that I am repeating something which the witness did not say, and doing it wilfully.

Mr Denniston: Oh, that was quite an exceptional instance.

Miss Houston (resuming) said: I was never away to pay visits during the time. I used not to sit with Captain Cain for any stated times, but I used to read to him often, and was daily in his room. When I first went to the house I used to read to him every evening, and after his illness I used to go into his room very often until Kay came, but was not in so often after that.

Mr Haggitt: Now I want you to describe how Captain Cain's illness progressed. You have had experience with sick people?

Witness: Not very much. I have been in a hospital nearly a year. I have not had much other experience with sick people. I had attended Mrs Matthias before I went to Captain Cain. I knew Captain Cain was suffering from dropsy, and that he had had gangrene a year or more beforehand.

You saw him daily. Did you notice changes taking place?

I could see he was getting gradually worse. I noticed he was more swollen every day and that his cough was worse, also that he got crosser and more irritable every day. He also got weaker. His appetite was very changeable. Sometimes he would eat lots of odds and ends of things in the course of a day and sometimes nothing. I think his appetite was always bad, because he used to tell us to get things for him which sometimes he used to eat and sometimes not. His sickness I think was very irregular. Sometimes he might be sick one day and not another day. I do not remember anything else. I did not notice anything that particularly made him sick. I often gave him his cough mixture, but never took notice what effect it had. I might have given it to to him and then left the room. I never saw him sick after taking the mixture. I have given him jellies, custards, and things and never seen him sick after them. He was sometimes fond of tea, but I do not remember him being sick after that. I do not know of any particular thing that made him sick. Bridget used principally to prepare his food. He used to have boiled fowl, chicken broth, jelly, oranges, and milk pudding sometimes. Sometimes we got things at his request which he did not eat. He used to have beef tea and mutton broth too. I think these things agreed with him.

Then what was it that made him sick?

Witness: I never could tell. I didn't take much notice of his sickness. I heard that he was always being sick.

And you never paid any attention to this ickness at all?

Witness: No. I never looked upon it as of any consequence. Nobody else seemed to think much of it, and I did not know much about it. Captain Cain gave up taking whisky before I went. While I was there he had champagne and wine and water. When he took his meals with me he used always to take wine and water—sometimes port and sometimes sherry. This was from September 1 to September 24. This wine was kept in a cupboard in the dining room. If I had known him to be sick I should not have put it down to the wine. I should have thought something had disagreed with him.

But if you noticed him sick after some particular thing?

Witness: He was not sick at any particular time. He was sick, I heard, after everything. I never observed that it was anything he drank, or anything in particular that made him sick. He had a cough and very bad feet. I don't think he had any pain in them, because he had no feeling at all.

Do you know of his complaining of thirst?

Oh, yes. He was always thirsty. My remembrance of him is that he was often drinking—generally wine and water and tea. He was always thirsty before and after Christmas.

Did that indicate anything to you?

Witness: I think people who have dropsy are always thirsty. If I thought about it at all, I should have put it down to dropsy. I did not know at the time that he suffered from diarrhœa. All the time he was very restless. He could not keep still when he could move about, and when he became unable to move someone had to move him. I think he was quite sensible and did not waken. When I spoke to him he always spoke sensibly to me. He would persist in having the room dark always.

Did you ever know him to fancy that he saw something?

Mr Denniston: That is rather a leading question.

Witness: I never noticed anything of the kind.

Mr Haggitt: Now, Miss Houston, take time in answering this question. I want you to tell us whether you ever nursed any other person who exhibited the same symptoms of sickness and thirst and was at the same time subject to diarrhœa?

Witness: No; I only nursed one other man with dropsy.

Mr Haggitt: But I asked you, any other person.

Mr Chapman: This is the question objected to. I do not know if it is a convenient time to raise the question which my learned friend has been hinting at several times, but when the time comes we wish to object.

His Honor: I suppose this is the time.

Mr Haggitt: I am going to ask such questions of this witness.

Mr Chapman: I object to it. Is it understood that we are to argue the point on this particular question?

His Honor: It is a question to which yes or no would be the proper answer, and there could be no objection to that; but if the witness says yes, another question will be put to her—Who was it?

Mr Haggitt: I will argue the general subject. We both know what we mean.

Mr Chapman: This evidence, I submit, is inadmissible, because it goes into matters outside the history of this case altogether, and into subjects not in existence at the time referred to by the evidence in this case, and into matters which should not be allowed to affect the issue now before the court, or the person now charged here. I rest my objection in the first instance on the ground that it touches upon matters irrelevant to this inquiry, and in fact wholly outside the history of this case.

His Honor: I have had occasion, Mr Chapman, to consider the cases very carefully. My own opinion is that up to a certain point at any rate the evidence proposed to be tendered is admissible. I think evidence would be admissible to show that some other person to whom the prisoner had access exhibited the same symptoms as Cain exhibited, and also to show that there was found in the excreta of such person the same substance as was found in Cain's body. I think the cases show that so far evidence is admissible. If, however, evidence is tendered to show that there was some motive for administering this drug to that other person, I confess to greater doubt. No doubt in one case evidence of the kind was admitted, but I am not altogether satisfied as to the reason of it. There is no doubt a difficulty. I admit the question of the admission of the whole of the evidence is not altogether without difficulty. There is the case, for instance, of the Queen against Winslow, where similar evidence was refused, and there has been no case where it has been decided except on circuit that such evidence is admissible. I shall admit the evidence at any rate up to the point I have indicated; whether I shall reserve the point for the decision of the court in *banc* is a question for my consideration ; that I need not settle now.

Mr Haggitt: As far as Regina v. Winslow is concerned the reasons are not given.

His Honor: No doubt; but there it stands.

Mr Haggitt: And as for there being no decision by the full court, there have been decisions by enough judges to constitute a full court.

Mr Chapman: But that is a very different thing; and those decisions are conflicting.

His Honor: I confess there is an element in the reasons in all the cases which I am not entirely able to follow. My opinion is that the evidence is admissible up to the point stated.

Mr Haggitt: I am prepared to take the risk of your Honor reserving the point.

His Honor: I think it ought to be in any case.

Witness continued: I had never before attended anyone who had symptoms similar to Captain Cain's. I know some of the symptoms which appeared during Mrs Hall's illness. She was sick and very sallow and weak. Sometimes she lost her appetite for a day or two, at other times it was very changeable. She had diarrhœa too. There were a great many more symptoms. She complained of itchiness in her eyes and pains in her stomach. I think the sickness was the worst sympton.

Mr Chapman again objected to the line of examination.

Witness: Prisoner, of course, lived in the same house. He gave her food to my knowledge. I know that at one period of her illness Mrs Hall was ordered ice water. I was not present when the prisoner gave her ice water to drink. I know that injections were ordered for Mrs Hall. The injections were beef tea, brandy, and pancreatine. I never saw these things used They were used by Mrs Ellison, the nurse. I on one occasion gave Mrs Hall some oysters to eat. I took them myself from the dining room, with a piece of thin bread and butter. The bread and butter was prepared by me. It struck me all at once that Mrs Hall would like some oysters, and I took them on the spur of the moment. Mr Hall and I used to dine alone at that time, but he had gone upstairs when I brought the oysters. Mrs Hall often fancied oysters, and I had taken them in to her before. This was the only occasion on which I took them from the dining room. I believe she was ill afterwards. It could not have been with the oysters, because they were perfectly wholesome. It must have been something else. Mrs Hall drank the iced water out of a wineglass. The ice was kept in the bath in the bathroom, and pieces broken off it when wanted. It was allowed to drain through muslin into a cup, and then poured into the wineglass. I have given her ice water myself prepared in this way. The ice water was ordered once. I used to go out sometimes from Woodlands to see Mrs Hall. Mrs Newton generally went with me. I did not go very often. The prisoner never drove me over. He often talked to me about Captain Cain. I used to talk to him, and he used to

talk to me too. Of course we were all interested in it. He once told me that he didn't think Captain Cain would ever get better, and that he was very ill. I don't remember anything else. I was often at Woodlands with Hall, Mrs Newton, Mrs Hall, and Miss Gillon. I don't remember Hall saying what the doctors ought to do to Cain. Hall was frequently at Woodlands. He came in the morning and also in the evening. He sat up with Captain Cain two half-nights. I got up between 1 and 2 and relieved him on these nights. They were two consecutive nights—I think after Christmas. I spent Christmas at Woodlands. It was very quiet, because Captain Cain was ill. I remember he came to dinner that day. I don't remember Hall being sick that day. The doctor came that day. I think Mr and Mrs Hall dined there that day. I only remember Hall being there two nights, but I can't remember when they were. I sat up a week with Captain Cain altogether. The reason we sat up with him was that he had to have his medicine and some food every few hours, by the doctor's orders. I did not sit up after Kay came. I was in house when Captain Cain died. I did not notice anything particular on the 28th, but I could see he was getting worse every day. I know nothing of invitations being sent out for a card party on the evening of the 28th. I do not remember Mr Meason being there on that evening. I have thought about it a good deal, and do not recollect anybody being there on the 28th. I went to bed about 11 o'clock, and was not disturbed during the night, but Mrs Newton was called up. I saw Captain Cain that morning about an hour before he died. Mrs Newton told her that she had been called up in the night, and that she thought her father was dying. I thought this could not be so, as he had been so often worse. I looked in and saw that he was dying. He was raised up in the patent bed, and was breathing in short gasps. He was quite quiet and otherwise was just as he had been. George Kay was there, so I did not stay. I did not see him again. About an hour after I had been into Captain Cain's room I heard the prisoner's buggy coming, and I went out on the verandah and told him I thought the captain was dying. Hall went into the captain's room, and came out about a minute or two afterwards and said that the captain was dead. After that Hall stayed a little time—not many minutes,—and then went into town to arrange about things, I think.

Cross-examined by Mr Denniston: I was present during the whole of Cain's illness and during the whole of Mrs Hall's illness. There was nothing in Mrs Hall's illness which made me think of Captain Cain's illness. When I took the oysters in to Mrs. Hall no person could have had the slightest idea that they were going to Mrs Hall. Nothing whatever was given with the oysters, except the bread and butter. The general opinion in the household was that Captain Cain would not recover, and the doctor expressed the same opinion. I did not think for a moment that the captain would recover. I expressed the opinion to Hall that Captain Cain would not recover. Hall always seemed to be sorry for Captain Cain. I remember Dr Macintyre saying to Mrs Newton in the drawing room that he could not tell how long the captain would live. I think he said he might live for days or for weeks. I went to Woodlands on the 1st of December. When I first went there Hall and Captain Cain were friendly, but not as friendly as they afterwards became. About the first week I was there, Cain would speak to Hall if he met him. The first time Hall stayed to a meal in the house was just before the captain was very ill. Captain Cain became ill shortly after I went to Woodlands, and from that time he exhibited the same symptoms, only the symptoms became worse. During Captain Cain's illness a large number of persons had access to him; they came and went as they chose. There was always liquor for old friends if they wanted it. The liquor was not locked up, but stood on the table, and the champagne, whisky, and brandy were open to them. Geo. Kay was not to take anything but port wine, and Mrs Newton thought we should get a cheaper wine for him. I do not remember anything unusual with Captain Cain after Hall had been sitting up half the night with him. Hall made hurried visits in the morning, but in the evening would stay about a quarter of an hour. I remember on one occasion Captain Cain was angry because Hall did not see him when he called, and I gave as an excuse that he (Captain Cain) was asleep when Hall called, and Hall did not wish to disturb him. After that Hall saw Captain Cain whenever he called. I became very friendly with Mrs Hall. A good deal of the Woodlands furniture was retained by Hall. I remember one of Mr Hall's dogs being ill two or three times. On one occasion something was wrong with one of the eyes of the dog, and Hall had a mixture to put in it. Once Hall complained that he had got some of the mixture in his own eye, and the result was that the pupil of the eye became dilated.

Re-examined by Mr Haggitt: I cannot remember the dates when the dog was ill, but it was after May 1886, before the dog was ill at Woodlands, and I remember it was ill before we went to Woodlands. I remember distinctly that on one occasion when Hall got some of this stuff into one eye. He put some morphia in his other eye, as an experiment, and the result was that it contracted the pupil of that eye. The mixture for the dog's eye was kept in a little cupboard in the bathroom at Woodlands, and there were a number of bottles in the same place. At Compstall they were kept on the bottom shelf in Mrs Hall's bedroom. There were a large number of bottles there, and some in the bathroom too. The contents of some of the bottles were connected with photography. I did not take notice of the bottles, and should not have known those connected with photography only I saw Mr Hall use them. Captain Cain was blind of one eye, and did not see very well with the other.

To Mr Denniston: The cupboards were quite open to any of them. I know the old dining room at Woodlands. Before the dining room was turned into a bedroom, the dining table stood at right angles with the fireplace, about the centre of the room. Anybody sitting at the head of the table could see into the cupboard if the doors were open.

To Mr Haggitt: The cupboard had double doors opening in the centre. Mrs Newton sat at the head of the table and Captain Cain sat opposite the window at the side of the table.

William Arthur Mason, agent for the National Mutual Life Insurance Association, Timaru, said: I knew the late Captain Cain very well indeed. I used to visit him very frequently,—as a rule in the evenings. To the best of my belief I was with him the night before he died. It was either that night or the one before. I cannot say I noticed any difference in him from the last time I had seen him. I stayed about a quarter of an hour with him. During the last fortnight of his life, was with him for a short time most evenings. I think on the last night I went by Mrs Newton's invitation to a card party. It was not only during the last fortnight of Cain's life that I was in the habit of dropping in of an evening. I used to for months before, and usually, but not always, sat with Captain Cain. He used to smoke while I was sitting with him, and I have seen him drink whisky. He complained to me that he could not drink whisky any longer. It was before the last fortnight of his life. He said it was strange that grog disagreed with him after he had taken it for 50 years. It made him sick, he said. I sometimes had whisky with him. I expect this was at the end of November or the beginning of December. I never saw him take the whisky anything but cold. I believe he took champagne when the grog disagreed with him. I have seen him taking cough mixture, but did not notice that it had any particular effect upon him. I have seen him sick, but did not attribute it positively to the cough mixture.

Cross-examined by Mr Chapman: I never saw him sick before his illness. It was gradual. In November I began to see that he was very poorly, and shortly after or about that time he began to be sick. Captain Cain was a very hospitable man. He used to ask me to have a glass of whisky or something else; or I used to take it without being asked. I knew him well enough for that.

Francis Worcester Stubbs, commission agent, Timaru, said: I knew the late Captain Cain, and sat up with him the night before he died. I first visited him after he became ill on the 13th January. He was in the dining-room sitting in an arm-chair, with his legs on other chairs. It was some time in the afternoon that I went. I gave him some champagne from a bottle on the sideboard. A syphon was in the bottle. The champagne agreed with him. On other occasions I have given him champagne, and have put the syphon into the bottle myself. A few days afterwards I gave him some, and that agreed with him too. I was there every day from January 13 to his death. The first few days I went in the afternoon, and after that I and Mr Buchanan took alternate nights to go and sit up with him. When I stayed there at night I went at about 8 o'clock in the evening. On one occasion I left at 1.30 a.m., and on other occasions stayed till 5 or 6 o'clock. Captain Cain never slept long together, and he always wanted something when he awoke. I gave him jelly, custards, and and champagne. The custards and jellies never seemed to disagree with him, and I never knew him sick after the champagne. I have seen him sick after taking whisky on two or three occasions, and I have seen him sick once or twice after taking medicine. I do not know what the medicine was. One afternoon he asked me to give him whisky, as he was tired of the champagne. I gave him some whisky out of an ordinary whisky bottle on the sidetable, and he was sick immediately after. A day or two afterwards he asked for more, and I gave him more whiskey out of the same bottle, and he was sick again. That was about the 18th and the 20th of December. At that time he was lying in the invalid bed. I remember that invalid bed coming. I was at the house the same afternoon. A r.an was sent to see about it, and brought a reply that it would be sent that evening. I saw Hall at the house the evening after the invalid bed came and asked Hall how he thought the captain was. Hall said he was very bad indeed, and could not get over it. I said I thought he was better than he was the day previous, and Hall said he did not think he could get through the night. I saw Hall at Woodlands on about three occasions only. The first time was previous to the invalid bed coming home, and then I think I saw him three or four days after the bed came. For some time Captain Cain appeared to me to get better. That continued for three or four days. Then for some days he remained about the same, then he became gradually weaker, but there was no sudden change until the night he died. I sat up with Captain Cain on the night he died. When I went there at 8 o'clock he appeared to be about the same, but a change came between half-past 12 and 2 o'clock. Kay and I sat up with him. I was with him all night. He had spells of sleep of about half-an-hour at a time, and at other times he talked to us. He talked about all sorts of things, and wanted to know what news was going in the town. He often talked about his sufferings, and wished he was away, but I could not say what he said on that particular night. He would talk perhaps for 10 minutes at the time. During that evening he talked about general topics. Then he would go to sleep again, and whenever he awoke he would ask for something, and wet his lips with champagne. I think too that he had some cough mixture. He would wake with a cough, and ask for the mixture. He went to sleep at from about half-past 9 or 10. Then he slept for an hour. After that he was taken up and his bed made comfortable. Either I or Kay gave him some champagne. He slept till about half-past twelve, when Kay and I were aroused by an alteration in his breathing. He generally breathed hard,

and the stoppage was so sudden that we both got up. He seemed peaceful. I caught hold of his pulse and found it slow and irregular. I got Kay to call Mrs Newton as I thought he was dying. Mrs Newton and Miss Gillon came down and Mrs Newton stayed for about an hour. The captain then suddenly started coughing and seemed to revive. He wanted to be taken up, and Mrs Newton left the room and he was taken up. He was then very weak, could not stand, and asked to be put down. We made him comfortable in bed, and he asked for more champagne and shortly went off to sleep again, but not into quite so peaceful a sleep as he was in before, but his breathing was not hard. He seemed to be comfortable, and sleeping nicely. He did not awake again before I left in the morning at 6 o'clock. I was afterwards told that he never awoke out of that sleep. I think he got his cough mixture early in the evening after I got there. So far as I can recollect he was not sick at all that evening. I do not know whether he suffered from diarrhœa.

To the Court : Captain Cain's face had quite changed in expression when we noticed the difference in his breathing. It looked peaceful and reposed.

The court adjourned at 5 30 p.m.

WEDNESDAY, JANUARY 26.

THIRD DAY OF THE TRIAL.

On the case being resumed at 10 a.m., The witness Stubbs was again put in the box and cross-examined by Mr Chapman. He said : I was at Woodlands on Tuesday night, January 26, and also on the 27th. I did not give Capt. Cain champagne; I got him some brandy. It made him sick every time he took it. It was no sooner in his mouth than it was out again. It was weak brandy and water. I asked for champagne and was told that there was none; that the doctor's instructions were that he was to have nothing but brandy. I saw Hall in the room three times. He only stayed a few minutes. I am not aware that Hall ever gave him anything in my presence. I saw Captain Cain vomit two or three times after giving him whisky. I never saw him sick after taking champagne. During the time I was attending Captain Cain I noticed some slight smell. His legs and the lower part of his body were very much swollen, and I was told he suffered from dropsy. I did not see Hall at Woodlands on January 26, 27, and 28. I last saw him there on the occasion of Wm. Newton's attempted suicide. His Honor : That date, if it is important, can be fixed by a file of the papers.

To Mr Haggitt : On January 26, 27, and 28 I only went into the sick room. Any number of persons might have been in the sick room without my knowledge.

John Kay deposed : I am a labourer. I attended on the late Captain Cain, commencing on January 1. Wren and I attended alternately. When I was on in the day Wren attended at night, and when I attended at night Wren came on in the day. Otherwise, I had only attended sick persons in my house. Hall came to Woodlands every day; sometimes more than once a day. I never stayed in the room while he was there. I used to go out because I understood he had business with the old captain. Prisoner has told me that he would stop with Cain for a few minutes. On one occasion he told me that he wished to speak to the captain for a few minutes, and that was quite sufficient for me. I sat up with the captain every night of the week he died. I did anything for him that he required. He was very restless, and wanted to get out of bed every 10 minutes. He was tired of his bed. As soon as he was got into bed and placed nice and comfortable he would want to be put up again. I used to sit alongside the bed or walk about. I never got any rest at all. When first I went he was very cheerful and chatty, but he was not quite so cheerful latterly. He never seemed to be in much pain. He slept occasionally for a quarter of an hour or 20 minutes—perhaps more. He would take these short sleeps pretty constantly. I used to give him his medicine during the night, also his food—chicken soup, lunch biscuits (when first I went there), and tea. He had very little food of any description during the last fortnight. The last week I gave him jelly only, so far as I can recollect. It agreed with him, but I cannot swear that he kept it down. Champagne was all that I gave him to drink. He "jibbed" on taking the cough mixture several times, saying it was nasty. There was another mixture from the doctor to abate the sickness. It was an effervescing drink, taken from two bottles and mixed. The cough mixture was all contained in one bottle. He took it when the cough was most troublesome. I believe I have given it him three times in a night. He was oftener sick after it than after anything else I have given him. I do not recollect his ever having been sick after the effervescing mixture. He was sick after his grog, and did not take a great deal of it during the month I was there. On one occasion we ran out of champagne, and I gave him brandy or whisky from the decanter. He was sick after taking it. Sometimes he kept the jellies down; sometimes he didn't. When first I went there I got him to smoke; he used to be in the habit of smoking before. He would take a few puffs and then put his pipe down. During the last week I did not notice any change in him until the night before his death. Sometimes he had looked better than at other times. On the night before his death I went on duty about 8 o'clock. He was restless and wanted to get out of bed at short intervals. He settled down after the change of death came on him, viz, after 1 o'clock. I believe he had some jelly that night, but cannot say whether he kept it down. There was no night that he was not sick very often—three or four times, or perhaps more. The sickness did not last long. He was sick more than once the last night. He had had champagne to drink; also the cough mixture. He repeatedly complained of the cough mixture being nasty, and refused to take it on several days. The first thing I noticed was a change in his features; he was in a doze. His breathing changed as

well, and I saw him move his body. (The witness drew himself out in order to show the attitude which the deceased assumed.)

Mr Haggitt: He stiffened himself?

Mr Denniston: He never used the word "stiffened." You have no right to put words into the witness' mouth.

Mr Haggitt: This is too much.

The Witness: I will not be induced to say anything but what took place.

Mr Denniston: We have perfect confidence in you, Mr Kay. It is the learned counsel's conduct that is objectionable.

Mr Haggitt: Really, this is intolerable.

Mr Denniston: It may be intolerable; but I say, when my learned friend puts the word "stiffened"——

Mr Haggitt: But the witness did stiffen himself. His attitude suggested the word.

Mr Denniston: But surely you have no right to put the words into his mouth.

His Honor: I cannot get the attitude of the witness on my notes. The attitude represented stiffness. I think it is quite legitimate. (To the witness): You made a gesture by stiffening yourself out.

Witness: It was a kind of twitching. Stiffening is what I meant. After this we saw him twitching now and again, but he never spoke again. This continued for some time. I noticed no change till 8 or 9 o'clock. He never seemed to alter. I awoke Mrs Newton, and she came into the room and remained a short while. Mr Stubbs went away early. I believe I called Denny (Wren) up afterwards. The deceased had diarrhœa some part of the time I was attending him; the latter part it was very severe. Sometimes I used to take tea when nursing the captain, and sometimes wine. I remember giving Jackson, the blacksmith, some champagne. This was on the day he brought home the bedstead. I took the champagne from a bottle which had been used for the captain. The bottle had been opened that day. In giving the captain champagne I used to strain it through muslin to prevent pieces of the cork coming into the glass. One day I was squalmish and sick. I do not know what I had taken that day. I am not accustomed to sickness, and have not been sick like it before or since. I have never seen Hall giving Captain Cain anything.

To Mr Denniston: I knew Captain Cain personally before I went to nurse him. I used to work for him.

Mr Denniston: He was very hospitable, wasn't he—not a stand-off sort of a man?

Witness: What do you mean—a man to "square up?"—(Laughter.)

Mr Denniston: A man who would easily make friends.

Witness: Yes, he was very friendly. He was not a man who would go to bed unless there was a good deal the matter with him. You may be sure he would not go to bed till he was absolutely compelled to. He suffered from dropsy. I know that there was a little water coming through his skin. One of his toes had been taken off about 18 months before, and there was a sore on one of his feet through a needle having run into it. It was on a Saturday that I was sick. I had been up all night with the captain, There was uot a very pleasant smell in the room sometimes. I had known the captain for 20 years. I don't know what made the captain change from wine to spirits. I can't remember details after such a long time. I got the jellies out of the pantry. Miss Houston and Mrs Newton used to be there—generally Miss Houston. Sometimes when a friend came to see the captain I used to take a turn round the verandah. I have no doubt his friends assisted him to anything be required while I was out.

Emma Ostler, a widow, residing at Timaru, deposed: I used frequently to visit the late Captain Cain's house. I very often dine l there. I recollect dining there in the early part of December 1885 at half-past 1. Captain Cain, Mrs Newton, Mr Hall, and I think somebody else were also present. Captain Cain said he was better before lunch. I went there about 11 o'clock. I asked him how he felt as I went in to dinner, and he said he felt better. During dinner he was asked to take whisky, and he refused, as, he said, it had begun to make him sick. I think it was Mrs Newton who asked him to take the whisky. Mr Hall then went to get him something else from the cupboard. He stooped down and poured something into a glass for him. He took Captain Cain's glass from the table. He was stooping down at the cupboard so that I could not see him pouring it into the glass, but I saw it in afterwards. The door of the cupboard prevented me from seeing his movements. He took the tumbler and put it by the side of Captain Cain, putting some water in it. When dinner was half over Captain Cain was very sick. We helped him from the room. I took one hand, and Hall went to get his bedroom ready. I don't know who was on the other side. I don't think I noticed any change in Captain Cain before this sickness came on. It came on very suddenly. I don't know what was in the glass. It was of a dark colour. During the latter part of Captain Cain's illness I was often at Woodlands I was twice at Hall's when Mrs Hall was so sick. I saw Mr Hall every time I was at Woodlands. I don't remember being there without seeing him. I have heard him say how sorry he was that the captain was in such pain, and ask wouldn't it be right of the doctors to give him something to ease it, and let him die quietly. This was three days before he died, when be was very ill indeed.

To Mr Denniston: I have known Captain Cain familiarly for 18 years. I knew Mr Brittain, a blood relation of his He was his youngest sister's son. Brittain was about 28. I knew him. He came on a visit to Captain Cain's, and stayed for a little while. The captain appeared very proud and fond of this young man. Mrs Hall and Mrs Newton were at Woodlands when he came. Mrs Hall was living there and Mrs Newton was on a visit. On the day that Captain Cain was taken ill t ere was whisky on the table. It was not an u ·usual thing to see it there. It was Captain Cain's refusal to take whisky that led to Mr Hall's getting him something else. Hall was sitting nearest to the cupboard. The captain was in great pain when Hall spoke about the doctor's giving him something.

Mr Denniston : I think he had expressed some such wish himself ?

Witness : I n ver heard him. I think he wanted to live very much.

Re-examined by Mr Haggitt: The witness detailed on a plan where the persons sat at dinner on the day she referred to. She continued : Captain Cain could hardly see at all. One eye was quite blind. I have seen him try to put the stopper in a decanter and he could hardly see the place where to put it. At the time of Mr Brittain's visit Mrs Hall was not married. It was on January 20, 1885, that Brittain came. It was not for a long visit

William Gunn, examined by Mr White, said : I am a chemist in Timaru. I know the prisoner. The book produced is an old sale of poisons book of mine dating from 1882 to 1886. On May 25 I see I made a sale of poison to T. Hall; it was of tartar emetic. The entry is " 5th May 1885. Mr Hall, Timaru, two drachms ant. tart., purposes medicinal ; signature, T. Hall." The entry is in my writing except the signature " T. Hall." On the 23rd of that month I lent Hall a mortar and pestle, also a 2oz measure and a set of scales. The measure was a graduated one from ½dr to 2oz The weights were from 1gr up to 2dr. These things were never returned to me. I have sold Mr Hall poison since then. I lent Hall the articles referred to on May 23, 1885. The next sale I made of poison was on June 18, 1886.

Mr Chapman said this was one of the questions he objected to, but he was not going to argue the question.

His Honor : Yes, this comes within the ruling I gave yesterday. I understand the point of your objection thoroughly.

Witness continued : The entry is 2 drachms tartar emetic to T. Hall, the prisoner. On the 26th of the same month there is an entry of 2dr tartar emetic and saltpetre. These were two different things. Accused said the cigarettes he made from the tartar emetic on the 28th were the best things he had ever bad for asthma, only they had one fault—they didn't burn well. Dr Lovegrove was there on the 26th, and I think he suggested the use of saltpetre. It was either he or I who suggested it. On July 5, 1886. there is an entry of 2oz colchicum wine to the accused. On the 17th July there is also an entry of 2oz colchicum wine ; on the 31st July a similar entry ; and on the 11th August another entry of the sale of the wine. I know these sales were made to the accused. All those entries are in my own handwriting.

To Mr Chapman: All these things were taken away from the shop by Hall, and I suppose they were kept by him. Hall had been an occasional customer of mine earlier than any of the dates mentioned. I think it was in 1892 that he came to deal with me. I used to make solutions for him for photographic purposes, but I never saw any specimens of his photography. I suggested that he should have the mortar, &c., as he always brought the pyrogalic acid and I had only to supply the bottle and some water. I suggested this to save myself trouble.

A pestle and mortar would be required to dissolve tartar emetic in cold water, but it dissolves very well in hot water. I have no recollection of any of Hall's purchases being returned. If such an unusual transaction as bringing back poison took place I would be sure to remember it, because I remember some transactions that took place on that day. About that time I began to oblige Hall by making solutions for photography. Hall said he had a receipt sent from John Shears from Loudon for making cigarettes from tartar emetic and stramonium seeds for asthma. I believe Hall was troubled with asthma, because he used to buy Joy's patent cigarettes. I believe he also suffered from sciatica. I sold him morphia for that. Colchicum wine is also good for sciatica. Tartar emetic is used as an expectorant, generally in the shape of antimonial wine. Most cough mixtures contain either antimonial wine or ipecacuanha wine, and it is a matter of opinion which is the better. Ayer's cherry pectoral is supposed to contain antimonial wine; the formula for it contains it at any rate. Cherry pectoral is not largely sold. It is sold by chemists, and also by storekeepers.

Re-examined by Mr White: Up to the 5th May 1885 Hall had only got prescriptions made up by order of Dr Lovegrove. It was since the prisoner's committal for trial that I have been asked about prisoner returning the tartar emetic. The managing clerk for the solicitors to the prisoner asked me concerning it.

Charles B. Eichbaum, a chemist in Timaru, said: On May 20, 1885, I sold an eyedropper and atropia eyedrops half an ounce. On Nov. 4, 1885, there is an entry in my assistant's handwriting. On June 3, 1886, there is an entry for 1oz of atropia that was sold by me to accused. On June 12 I sold antimonial wine 2oz. On July 6, tincture of colchicum 1oz, and 2oz wine of colchicum. The tincture was returned to me. On August 4, 1886, there is an entry for stramonium seeds, nitrate of potash, and half an ounce of tartar emetic. Accounts of all these sales were rendered to the prisoner up to June 30, and no objection was made by him.

To Mr Denniston : Atropia eyedrops are very commonly used. In March it was an original prescription by Dr Hogg.

Mr Haggitt: That was for the foal.

Mr Denniston: My dear sir, you don't know what it was for yet; you've not proved it.

Mr Haggitt: But we shall.

Witness continued: Nitrate of potash is saltpetre. Colchicum wine is a good specific for rheumatism.

Joseph John Heskins, a chemist's assistant, living in Dunedin at present, deposed: In 1885 and 1886 I was an assistant to Mr Eichbaum in Timaru. There is an entry in my handwriting for November 4 for a sale of atropia to Hall. On January 28, 1886, there is an entry made by me for eyedrops. I remember the sale of that. The eyedrops consisted of a solution of atropia, half an ounce. There were four grains of atropia to the ounce in each solution.

To Mr Chapman: It was the ordinary pharmacopœa strength that I used. It is sometimes used still further diluted. Hall said at the time

that he was using it for one of his animals. He came from his office for it.

Roderick Fraser Stewart was the first witness called after the luncheon adjournment. He said that he was a chemist in the employ of Mrs Watkins at Timaru. On November 13, 1885, there was an entry of wine of colchicum (2oz) sold to the prisoner.

William Henry Willway, accountant to Mrs Watkins, said that in the year 1885 prisoner had an account with Mrs Watkins. The wine of colchicum spoken of by the last witness was paid for by the prisoner.

William Henry Trilford, groom, living at Timaru, was formerly in the prisoner's service. This was before Captain Cain's death. John Wilson followed him in the prisoner's service. He (witness) left just after Christmas, 1885. Hall had a foal which got its eye hurt with a barbed wire. The foal got its eye hurt shortly after Hall married. Another horse which had something wrong with its mouth was sent down to Harry Gardener's, at Saltwater creek.

To Mr Chapman: There was something the matter with the eyes of one of Hall's dogs.

Harry Gardener, licensee of the Sportsmans' Arms Hotel, Saltwater creek, near Timaru, stated that in 1885 he treated a horse for Hall. It was suffering from influenza. To the best of his belief this would be in November. He steamed its head with hot bran. Neither of its eyes was affected.

To Mr Denniston: Influenza would lead to a slight affection of the eyes.

John Wilson : I am an apprentice to a painter in Timaru. In January 1886 I entered the employment of the prisoner. There were ferrets, horses, and dogs about the place. I don't know that there was anything wrong with those animals. Two cats died.

Mr White : Did they die suddenly ?

Mr Denniston : Oh, really, are we to have an inquiry about the death of the cats?—(Laughter)

Mr White : Was there anything unusual about their death ?

Witness : No. One died about a week after the other.

Peter William Hutton, bookseller and stationer in Timaru, said: I have been resident in Timaru for 20 years. I have seen the book " Headland's Action of Medicines " produced before. I sold it to the prisoner in May 1885. On looking at my daybook I find the entry of the sale is on the 9th May 1885. I saw the prisoner come into the shop while I was serving a customer and go round to where the medical books are kept. I went round and said "Good day, Mr Hall." He asked, " Have you any book treating on the subject of antimony?" I took down this volume, and referring to the contents found a chapter on antimony, which I turned up. The leaves being uncut, I held the book open, and said, " Here, Mr Hall, is the chapter you are inquiring for." With my permission, a few of the leaves treating of that subject were cut and the book purchased. Prisoner took it with him. Pages 371 to 375 were cut—the chapter treating of antimony. The chapter on neurotics I also found cut—pages 273 to 296. I now find no other leaves cut. I recognise the other book produced—"Taylor on Poisons." It belonged to me. The prisoner had returned "Headland's Action of Medicines," and about a month afterwards I found him up in the medical corner of the shop again. He asked me if I would have any objection to lend him "Taylor on Poisons," and I said certainly not if he took care of it. This was on a Saturday about June, and he brought it back on the Monday. A week or a fortnight afterwards he borrowed it again and kept it about the same time. On his returning it the second time I made the remark, "Mr Hall, you had better purchase this book. I have had it a considerable time in stock and I will make it cheap." I told him the price—16s 6d, I think—and he paid or it in cash, saying "You had better not book this." He was 3s short, and he sent that down afterwards. He took the book away with him. He first opened the book and wrote something in pencil at both ends of it. I find now written at the beginning, "T. Hall, 1882," and at the end, "T. Hall, Dunedin, 1882." It was not in 1882 or in Dunedin that I sold it to him. The writing is very like the prisoner's.

Mr Denniston (rising to cross-examine) : Have you got a good memory ?

Witness: Well, I am mortal.

But you can turn on a mental tap and remember things, can you not ? You have a special memory ?

I think I have for special things, also general things. It depends whether the things are worth remembering.

Have you told us all that took place ?

I have not been asked.

Oh, but it is not our business to ask you. That is for the Crown.

Witness : I will tell you more if you ask me.

Mr Denniston : Indeed. Then you have not told us all ?

Witness : After he paid for the book there was a conversation between us, principally on the subject of books on poisons. Hall was asking if I had any in stock. I never told this in examination in any other court.

Mr Denniston : Is not that very striking ?

Witness : No. I wished to do nothing to prejudice the prisoner.

Mr Denniston : Is there any other trifle ?

Well, I have not finished that yet. I said, "No, I have none of those books," and felt a little annoyed at his asking for them. I said, "If you want books on poisons, Mr Hall, I will order them for you in England."

For what reason were you a little annoyed ?

It was such a singular thing for a citizen to come in and ask for such things that it left a very unfavourable impression on me, and it still does, and always will.

Mr Denniston : No doubt, and we shall hear of it to your dying day. Hall, you say, asked if you had any books treating of antimony. Was that all he said ?

Witness (pointing to the depositions in counsel's hand) : You will find it there.

Was that all he said ?

You will find it there.

Was that all he said ?

You will find it there.

After this question and answer had been repeated some half-dozen times amidst laughter in court, the witness said,

As far as my memory serves, that is all Hall said.

Did he not pass his hands down his legs in this fashion and say, "You know what I suffer from" ?

Yes.

How is it you did not tell us this, then ?

I have not read over my evidence.

Because it is a circumstance we consider a little favourable to the prisoner, you know. It did not occur to you ?

No. If it had come into my mind I should have mentioned it. I do not attach any particular interest to the subject. I have no feeling against Hall.

Indeed. Did you not have a little row ?

Yes, we did. Would you like it retold ?

Oh, certainly ; as much as you can remember without reading over your evidence.

Well, are you ready for me to begin ?

I have been ready for some time, Mr Hutton.

Well, Hall came into the shop one evening and was in the act of purchasing a book, "King Solomon's Mines," and in the course of wrapping up the book I made the remark, "Have you heard from Mrs Newton yet ?" meaning in reference to the account she owed me. Hall said, "No ; but I would not advise her to pay it." The account was for goods supplied, part being for marriage presents to prisoner's wife and the rest for school books, and I made the remark that had she explained her position to me, as you would expect a lady to do, I should at once have made a reduction. But she refused a discount, put up her cheque-book, and went out of the shop like a duchess with £20,000 a-year.—(Laughter.) Hall then at once made use of the expression, "Damn the ladies !"

Mr Denniston : Are you sure he did not say "Damn the duchesses" ?

Witness : I said I would not allow an expression of that sort in the building, and if he used such an expression I had only one alternative, viz., to say "Damn the gentlemen."—(Great laughter.) Hall at once threw down a book on the counter and said, "Send in your account to-morrow, Mr Hutton." I said, "Certainly," and the account was sent in and paid.

Mr Denniston : You have sworn to the identity of this book (Taylor on Poisons); will you be good enough to tell me the special marks by which you identify it ?

Witness pointed to a portion of the cover that was very considerably frayed.

Mr Denniston : Do you mean to swear that is how you identify the book—that that mark was there when it was in your possession ?

Witness : I have not sworn——

Mr Denniston : What do you mean by pointing out that to the jury ?

Witness : How dare you tell me——

Mr Denniston : Oh, I dare tell you a great deal.

Witness : I knew that mark was there when I sold the book, although I did not look to see if it was. I swear it is the book.

You swear that mark was on it when you sold it though you did not notice it?
I have noticed it for five or six years.
Is that your answer?
Just allow me.
You have told the jury you knew that mark was on the book although you did not see it when you sold it. Do you mean that?
I may have said so.
Do you mean it?
It doesn't affect the evidence.
The jury will judge of that. Did you tell them a few minutes ago that mark was on the book when you sold it although you did not notice it?
My evidence has not been taken down.
And you would prefer it slightly altered?
That mark was on the book when I sold it. You swear it?
Yes.
You swear you carried in your memory that mark? Would any reasonable treatment in your shop cause such a mark on the book?
Yes. It was shifted from shelf to shelf.
To which shelf was it shifted?
I cannot tell you without a plan.
When was it you first noticed this mark—years or months before you sold the book?
I cannot tell. I swear to the book.
You swear you mentally identify it as having that mark at the bottom of the cover without looking at it. Tell us another book in your stock that is ear-marked.
Witness: Keep your temper, and I will keep mine.
Mr Denniston: I never was farther from losing my temper, I assure you, Mr Hutton. Do you want the jury to believe that out of 2000 books you carried the mark on this one in your memory?
The jury will judge of that.
I hope so. Is there any other mark on it?
There is a faint indication of my private mark, " H.I., —— U.", and the selling mark, " 18—6." But I will swear to the book. When I sold it was in much about the same condition as now.
Mr Denniston (holding up some loose leaves): Was it like this?
Witness: I could not say.
Mr Haggitt: But you still swear positively it is the book you sold?
Witness: I do most solemnly swear it.
Patrick Macintyre, medical practitioner at Timaru, said: I attended the late Captain Cain for many years, and during his last illness. This extended over about six months; I attended him almost daily from 1st January. I attended him in December too, pretty frequently. I attended him from 17th December to 28th January daily, with the exception of one day in January. In the early part of his illness I was attending him for general debility, feeble action of the heart, and senile gangrene. The gangrene sores healed up; the stump of the right little toe also healed up. This took place about 18 months before his death. He improved considerably after this, but about six months before his death he again got ill and became very weak. This was in July 1885. I attended him at intervals from that time until 17th December, when my attendance became constant. In July I attended him twice—on the 9th and 10th—for general debility. I prescribed for him on the 10th a tonic and stimulating mixture. I did not see him again till the 31st August, when I did not prescribe for him. I have no doubt I saw him then for his general weakness. On 5th September I prescribed for him a diuretic and cough mixture. The latter contained carbonate of ammonia, tincture of squills, spirits of chloroform, syrup of orange, and an infusion of senega. I do not know how long he continued to take this. On November 3 I prescribed an effervescing mixture to relieve sickness probably. It consisted of bicarbonate of potash and bicarbonate of soda, and dilute prussic acid and tartaric acid; I had half-drachm doses of extract of ergot added to this as a stimulant to the kidneys. I have no record of prescribing on 7th November. During this time from 9th July to 7th November, I was treating him for chest affection and dropsy. The dropsy was consequent upon congestion of the kidneys and heart affection. My next prescription was on 18th December, and contained sweet spirits of nitre, potassium, syrup of orange, chloric ether, and an infusion of uvae ursi to act on the kidneys. This was a diuretic. On 21st December I prescribed carbonate of ammonia, compound tincture of lavender, syrup of orange, chloric ether, and water. This was a stimulating mixture—more directly stimulating than a tonic. I don't know how long he continued to take this. On the 24th December I prescribed the effervescing mixture as before without the extract of ergot. On 27th December I prescribed compound spirits of ammonia, sweet spirits of nitre, syrup of orange, tincture of cinchona, and water. This was a tonic and stimulant. On December 30 I prescribed gall and opium ointment, with vaseline ointment added, for a sore in the foot, the result of gangrene. On 2nd January 1886 I prescribed bicarbonate of potash, nitrate of potash, liquor taraxacum, syrup of orange, compound tincture of lavender, and an infusion of uvae ursi. This was as a diuretic and a tonic to the liver. On 6th January I prescribed tincture of catechu, tincture of kino, a sedative, preparation of opium and chalk mixture. This was for diarrhœa. On 9th January, vaseline ointment for the foot; on 13th January, carbonate of ammonia, solution of acetate of ammonia, camphor mixture, syrup of orange, and water. He continued to take the effervescing mixture and cough mixture at intervals to the time of his death. I omitted one prescription of 18th January—compound spirits of ammonia, tincture of cinchona, chloric ether, syrup of orange, and water. There was also a stimulating mixture in June 1885, and there were other prescriptions in 1884. The cough mixture he took up to the time of his death was the same as one prescribed for him in his 1884 illness. It consisted of carbonate of ammonia, chlorodyne, compound tincture of camphor, syrup of squills, sweet spirits of nitre, and an infusion of senega. He at one time took it regularly, and I finally ordered that he

should be allowed to have it whenever his cough was troublesome. There was nothing in that mixture likely, in my opinion, to produce sickness. It ought not to produce sickness in a person in the state of health in which Captain Cain was at the last. There was no nasty taste. The flavour would be pleasant and sweetish. The other mixture he took down to the end was the effervescing mixture to relieve sickness and vomiting. That was not likely to make him sick, and there was nothing nasty in it. I am not aware that he was taking any other medicine during the latter part of his life. On 24th December 1885 I first heard of his being troubled with sickness. In November I prescribed the effervescing mixture for a feeling of sickness, but the first I knew of actual vomiting was on 24th December, and I then repeated the mixture without the extract of ergot Captain Cain complained to me of his inability to take whisky. I do not know the exact date. He said it tasted nasty, and he could not take it. I prescribed wines and brandy from time to time. He only once complained about the whisky. I believe he told me it made him sick. I do not remember whether it was before he took to his bed that he stopped the whisky. I continued to treat him for the general debility, dropsy, kidney disease, and cough up to the time of his death. There was weak action of the heart, which must have been of long continuance. I first knew of that when he took ill 18 months before his death. The heart disease was the cause of the kidney disease, in my opinion. The disease of the vessels and the impaired action of the heart caused the arrest of the circulation in those places where the gangrene came. It caused congestion of the kidneys, and it was principally this that produced dropsy, aided by feeble heart action. The dropsy and kidney disease never improved. Captain Cain was suffering from diarrhœa, and complained of being sick very often. These symptoms do not always occur in such disease. They may both occur. I was aware he suffered from thirst. This is not a very marked symptom of kidney disease and dropsy. Latterly the symptoms continued the same with increasing weakness. From the beginning of his illness in July he gradually went from bad to worse. On 28th January, in the afternoon or evening, I saw him last. He was very prostrate, breathing heavily and inclined to be very sleepy. On speaking to him he was with difficulty aroused, and then would lapse into slumber. This continued all the time I was there that day, and I did not see him again before his death on the following morning. I certified disease of the kidneys and dropsy as the cause of death. I returned his age as about 70 years. I attended Captain Cain's funeral. He was buried in the Timaru cemetery on 31st January. At the time I gave the certificate I believed it to be correct. Something occurred after the 15th August that caused me to think further on the subject of Captain Cain's death. He died at Woodlands, and after his death Hall and Mrs Hall went to live there. I attended Mrs Hall at her confinement in June 1886. She began to vomit about four days after her confinement.

Mr Chapman : I suppose it is not necessary for me to take a formal objection to this evidence?

His Honor : No ; the same objection covers it.

Witness : This vomiting and also purging continued for a period of about two months. She became gradually weaker, and finally on the 15th August she was in a state of c llapse when I calle l at the house. She had a nurse—Mrs Ellison— n attendance upon her. There w re intermissions and remissions in the sickness. She complained of a hot, burning feeling in the gullet, a feeling of constriction in the throat, and a pain in the pit of the stomach gradually extending over the whole of the abdominal region. There was a yellow jaundiced colour of the skin just before and during sickness. The lips were dry a d tender. At one period the tongue was unduly re l round the edges. There was great itching of the skin. The eyelids and nostrils were irritable. She had twitchings of the arms. The vomiting was sometime mucous, and sometimes mucous and bilious matter mixed. There was thirst. I did not discover the cause of these symptoms until it occurred to me to make a certain analysis on 15th August. Two or three days before that I examined some urine and vomit by Renisch's test. I got a violet deposit on the copper, which I believed to be antimony. I preserved a portion of each liquid, and sent them to Professor Black. While awaiting the result of his analysis Mrs Hall told me on visiting her——

Mr Chapman : This is a very long way from the subject of this inquiry.

Witness : I was informed of something by Mrs Hall and the nurse, and in consequence of this I took possession of some ice water handed me by the nurse. I had prescribed ice several days before for Mrs Hall's use, and given instructions as to the mode of its preparation. I analysed a portion of the ice water given me by the nurse the same day, and found antimony. The other portion I sealed up, and handed to Inspector Broham that Sunday night —the 15th August Dr Drew assisted me in the analysis of the ice water. The arrest of Hall followed.

Mr Chapman : That is not evidence.

Mr Denniston : How can he prove that?

Mr Haggitt : I want you to follow on the condition of Mrs Hall.

Witness : She underwent steady improvement from that date. The prisoner had prior to this been in attendance on his wife, and after this Sunday he ceased to be in attendance upon her. She kept on mending. I made further experiments after this on the urine and obtained indications of antimony by degrees passing out of the system. The traces got less daily. I followed up the examination for five days or a week after the arrest, and Dr Black and Dr Ogston took it up from that time. I supplied them with the excreta which was handed me by the nurse. All symptoms of antimony in Mrs Hall have now disappeared. It was after this occurrence that my attention was attracted again to the subject of Captain Cain's death. The sickness, vomiting, and purging attracted my attention, and I in conjunction with others took such steps that the body of Captain Cain was exhumed. I was present at the exhumation and saw the body, but took no part in the exhumation or the *post mortem.* Dr Ogston and Dr Hogg performed the *post mortem,* and I saw them cut away portions of the body, put it in bottles and take away. I accompanied them to Dunedin, and was present at the university during the time a portion of the analysis was being made.

Mr Haggitt : Now, what is the effect of antimony upon the human system ?

Witness : It is an irritant and a depressent. It causes burning pain at the throat, gullet, and stomach—the pain generally extending over the bowels—sickness, vomiting, and purging, extreme depression generally ending in death. The symptoms vary in different cases. The quantity administered and the age and condition of the patient affects the symptoms. Antimony is more likely to prove fatal in small than in large doses, because the stomach more readily rejects large doses.

What would be the likely effect of repeated small doses of antimony administered to a person suffering from kidney disease and dropsy ?

It would increase the depression already existing, and would sooner or later aid in bringing about the death of the patient.

What would be the case if in addition to kidney disease and dropsy there was also affection of the heart?

There would be still greater danger.

Supposing antimony in small doses to have been administered to Captain Cain during the last fortnight of his life, what effect would it have had ?

I consider it would have hastened his death.

What quantity to a person in his state would have been sufficient in your opinion ?

Witness : In one dose two grains have killed, and might very possibly have killed him. A continuation of two-grain doses would be certain to kill if continued long enough. When antimony does not kill at once it exercises a depressing effect on the heart. There is a lowering of the vital powers, and the person to whom it is administered ultimately succumbs from exhaustion and inability to retain food. Nausea, vomiting, depression, increasing weakness, and diarrhœa—symptoms of antimony poisoning—were present in Captain Cain's case. The diarrhœa from antimony poisoning is not continuous always ; it sometimes alter nates with constipation. I am not quite certain if Captain Cain's diarrhœa was continuous. I know he suffered from constipation either before or after the diarrhœa came on. The pulse in antimony poisoning becomes frequent and feeble. It was so in Captain Cain's case.

Colchicum is also a poison, is it not ?

Yes. The symptoms it produces are very similar to antimonial poisoning. It is a vegetable poison. A poison of that kind is not traceable in the system after death. It disappears probably in a few days or perhaps in a few hours. After a period of eight months it would be useless to look for it.

What is the effect of another poison, atropia ?

It causes a dryness and burning in the throat, first excitement of the nervous system, followed by delirium and stupor. It causes dilation of the pupils. The other symptoms are vomiting and nausea. Atropia is also a vegetable poison, and I do not consider it to be traceable at all after death. Antimony, on the other hand, is a mineral poison, and can be traced a long time after death. Neither antimony, colchicum, or atropia entered into any of my prescriptions, and antimony cannot be the result of decomposition of the human body. My prescriptions were made up at Watkins' dispensary at Timaru.

During your attendance upon Captain Cain, did you ever see Hall at Woodlands?

I have no distinct recollection of seeing him there. I remember him on one occasion talking to me about Captain Cain's condition. He inquired, I think, as to the probable course of the captain's illness, and how long he was likely to live. I am not aware that he suffered any great pain.

The court at this stage (5.10 p.m.) adjourned, Mr Chapman saying that it would be more convenient to go on with the cross-examination the following day. He would probably be able to save the time of the jury by doing so.

THURSDAY, JANUARY 27.

FOURTH DAY OF THE TRIAL.

Thomas Hall was again placed in the dock upon the charge that he, on the 9th January 1886, did feloniously, wilfully, and with malice aforethought, kill and murder one Henry Cain.

Mr B. C. Haggitt (Crown prosecutor at Dunedin), assisted by Mr White (Crown prosecutor at Timaru), appeared for the Crown ; Mr F. R. Chapman, with him Mr J. E. Denniston (instructed by Mr Perry, of Timaru) for the defence.

The case was resumed at 10 a.m.

Dr Macmtyre (cross-examination by Mr Chapman continued) : Captain Cain in his illness 18 months before his death lost a toe. That was attributed to a senile gangrene—a state of decay in a person still living. I attribute it to heart disease and disease of the artery. I cannot say whether the loss of the toe might be connected with diabetes. I never examined for diabetes in Cain's case. I examined for heart disease. There is not necessarily any connection between diabetes with Bright's disease, but when a man has diabetes Bright's disease of the kidneys may follow upon it. Congestion or Bright's disease may be associated with diabetes. I examined Cain's chest and satisfied myself of the presence of heart disease. That was from 18 months to two years prior to his death. I certified that Cain died from kidney disease and dropsy, and did not specify heart disease. Captain Cain suffered from chronic congestion of the kidneys, not from Bright's disease. According to the old nomenclature, all kidney diseases were called Bright's disease, and according to the nomenclature of the present day several kidney diseases all called Bright's disease. The detection of albumen in the r—i · · · a ʺfʹcult process. In Bright's disease you would find tube casts, and probably blood cells in the urine. I do not think Cain suffered from Bright's disease but from simple congestion, arising from heart disease. In the lower court I spoke of it as Bright's disease, classifying it under the old classification, in which all or nearly all diseases of the kidneys with albumen were called Bright's disease. There are three forms of kidney disease new classified as Bright's disease. Besides these you might have cancerous disease of the kidney, stone of the kidney, or tumor of any kind, which are not classified as Bright's disease, but probably would previously have been so classified. I was not aware of the more recent classification when I was examined in the court below. Eighteen months or two years before Cain's death I tested the urine and found it albuminous. My change of expression is due to subsequent reading. I do not think a stimulating diuretic would have the effect of increasing congestion in chronic congestion of the kidneys; but I would not say positively that it might not. I added ergot to another prescription to stimulate the muscular action of the kidneys. Captain Cain during the last six months was troubled with a cough, and I see that I prescribed for him for a cold in 1884. I then prescribed a cough mixture. After the appearance of bronchitis I noticed dropsy, and prescribed for it. The prescription of the 5th September is the first that would point to the existence of dropsy. I used to converse pretty freely with Captain Cain as to what was the matter with him, but have no distinct recollection of informing other members of the family from time to time of what was the condition of Captain Cain, though I probably did so. I used to meet Mrs Newton and Mrs Hall, and might have told them of the nature of the disease. I can remember one occasion on which I told them that Captain Cain might die at any moment, or live for weeks or months. From the time Captain Cain took ill in July I always regarded it as a case in which that disease would end in death. I felt pretty sure that he would die of the diseases from which he was then suffering, and I did not disguise that fact from the family. My conclusion that he would die of his diseases was not altered by discovering on the 5th of September that he was suffering from dropsy. The discovery of dropsy would be a strong confirmation of my opinion that he was labouring under disease which would prove fatal. Senile gangrene is recognised as the result of kidney disease, Bright's disease, and diabetes. Senile gangrene in itself is a cause of fatal exhaustion of the whole system, and is sometimes, or even frequently, a source of blood poisoning. Pain was not a feature of Cain's case. That circumstance is strongly consistent with the diseases he was suffering from; he might suffer from those diseases and die of them without experiencing much pain. All those diseases taken together indicate a case of senile break-up and decay. It is rather characteristic of a case like Cain's that the diseases should run their course and the patient die without suffering marked pain. In a declining case of that sort I should not be surprised at finding diarrhœa. If Cain had not been stimulated freely

he would have died more readily from the diarrhœa alone, considering that he suffered from other diseases. Over-stimulation does in some cases provoke diarrhœa; and in a particular person one form of stimulant may produce diarrhœa when another will not. I did not order stimulants to the extent of four quart bottles of champagne a day. I did not specify the quantity; but he might have been allowed from one pint bottle up to two pint bottles in the 24 hours, as well as a little stronger stimulant occasionally. At first the quantity of cough mixture was limited by the direction on the bottle, and subsequently I removed the limitation because I thought less was required. I directed it to be taken when the cough was troublesome. The medicine went in 8oz bottles, and a bottle should have lasted from two to four days. The cough mixture contained morphia, opium, and ammonia. This medicine taken in large quantities might cause the patient to take a great dislike to it; and if taken with a larger amount of stimulant than was intended, it might produce a great deal of thirst. If taken on any particular day in excessive quantities it might produce nausea and vomiting. It would probably cause irritation of the stomach prior to vomiting, but I do not think the irritations would extend far from the stomach. I should expect it, if retained, to produce constipation. I cannot say it would not produce purging. It is characteristic of an opiate, if there is too much of it or if the circumstances are not favourable, that it should produce nausea and vomiting. In people who are ill we find all sorts of idiosyncrasies of taste and apparent caprice. In small quantities tartar emetic in solution is tasteless. I have not had much to do with Bright's disease. It is the case that both diarrhœa and sickness may be characteristic of the diseases from which Cain suffered. Thirst is also quite consistent with the diseases from which Cain suffered. I never really hoped for a recovery in Cain's case. It was characteristic of the diseases from which he was suffering that I should find him near the end in the drowsy state in which I found him on the 28th of January. That condition is due to the effect of something upon the brain. The kidneys ceasing to act and carry off the waste of the body, that waste is retained in the blood and acts on the brain—a kind of blood-poisoning is produced which affects the brain. This is called urine poisoning, and it affects a good many old people. It was in the afternoon or evening of the 28th January that I saw Captain Cain. I do not remember the hour. The twitching about the face is quite possible as a symptom of urine poisoning, and is characteristic of the final stage of many diseases. In treating dropsy, free purging by active drugs is frequently resorted to, and these may cause vomiting. These drugs are beneficial if there is no vomiting, but vomiting would induce me to discontinue their use. I noticed certain symptoms in Mrs Hall's case four days after her confinement. Mrs Hall was a strong, robust woman and had had a healthy and normal confinement. Her peculiar symptoms attracted my attention at once. These symptoms were sickness and vomiting, and were quite inconsistent with her condition. I ultimately ascertained to my satisfaction what she suffered from, and from the 15th of August onward she progressed steadily to recovery, though she suffered depressing effects for some months afterwards. Before last year I had no actual experience of antimonial poisoning. If one of my answers yesterday was that the age and the condition of the patient affected the symptoms, I wish to correct that by saying they do not. After a large dose of antimony the whole or nearly all the poison would be rejected. A person has recovered after taking 468 grains in a dose. It is possible that in one remarkable case in which a large quantity of antimony was taken, mustard had to be administered to produce vomiting. When speaking of large doses I was not speaking of ounce doses. From 15 to 20 grains have been taken by people without producing disastrous results. Very large doses amounting from 15 to 30 grains are reported to have been given, and I presume repeated in the treatment of certain cases. Antimony has been found to be extremely variable in its effects, judging from recorded cases. I have met with no case in which a person suffering from the diseases from which Cain suffered has taken antimony, and have no actual knowledge of its effect upon such cases. Since this case cropped up I have read a good deal about antimony in standard works, and according to them it produces widely different effects on different persons.

Mr Chapman : Is it not the case, looking at the extreme variation of results in recorded cases, that it is very much a matter of speculation what effect it would produce on a given individual ?

Witness : When given in acute inflammatory diseases the patient can tolerate very much more than a healthy person could. That is also the case with aconite in fever cases. The symptoms produced by antimony are pretty well known.

Mr Chapman : But supposing you had the opportunity to experiment upon those 12 gentlemen, and gave them all the same dose, is it not the case that it would produce varying effects upon different individuals ?

Witness : I should say it is only a matter of degree, provided they got the same dose. The use of antimony in medicine is a matter over which medical authorities at different dates have differed widely. I believe there are some who even to this day prescribe antimony freely, but they are comparatively few. It is the congestive kind of kidney disease that generally accompanies heart disease. I never noticed any offensive smell in Captain Cain's room. The room was particularly well ventilated. The nurses might have experienced an offensive smell though I did not.

RE-EXAMINED.

Mr Haggitt: Has anything you have been asked to-day altered the opinion you expressed yesterday as to the effect of a small dose of antimony administered to a person in the condition Captain Cain was during his life ?—No.

Although it may be a fact that under certain circumstances antimony may be administered without actually causing harm, if a person has heart disease, coupled with kidney disease and dropsy, I understand you to say that it could not be administered to him without causing harm ?—It could not be.

Witness (examination resumed) : The effect of antimony upon a person suffering from those diseases would be to cause great depression and to accelerate death. The cases in which antimony has been administered without injury have been cases of inflammatory fever. The age of a patient does not affect the symptoms in a case of antimonial poisoning, I should say ; that is to say, the symptoms in a child would not be different from the symptoms in an adult, but an old and diseased person would succumb before all the symptoms which would occur in a healthy person would show themselves. It is dangerous under any circumstances to administer antimony to an old person, and it is recognised that it must not be given even medicinally to an old person. No medical man prescribed for Captain Cain except myself. I never prescribed antimony for him. There were about 2½ dracms of chlorodyne in the 8oz bottle, and the quantity of morphia in that would be very small. There would be about the 15th of a grain of opium in each dose, and 16 doses in the bottle. One grain of opium might make a man in Captain Cain's condition sick—from one to three grains would ; and there would not be quite a grain of opium in the whole bottle. At one time I ordered that Captain Cain should have nothing but champagne, as he could not retain food. I intended that he should have at that time about a quart a day, and he was allowed a little other stimulants as well. If he took nothing but champagne he would probably he allowed a little more than a quart a day. Senile gangrene was not a cause of fatal exhaustion in Captain Cain. The captain had suffered from gangrene 18 months before, but it had healed up, and only one gangrenous spot broke out during the last illness. Pain was not a feature of Captain Cain's case, and pain is a feature of Bright's disease, and towards the end the pain sometimes became intense. I told Captain Cain he had dropsy, but do not remember telling him he had kidney disease. I think I told Captain Cain at Watkins' chemist shop that he was suffering from dropsy, but I do not remember the date.

To Mr Chapman : I may have conversed with Captain Cain about his dropsy more than once, but I cannot remember doing so. I may have told other members of the family that the captain had dropsy. Acute pain is not common in Bright's disease, but a certain amount of dull aching pain across the back may be said to be characteristic of it.

Dr Drew (a medical practitioner and surgeon, residing at Timaru), examined by Mr Haggitt, deposed : I am surgeon at the Timaru Hospital. I knew Captain Cain personally and some of his friends intimately. I saw Captain Cain on the 28th of January, the day before he died. I called simply as a friend to see him. Captain Cain was sitting up in bed. He seemed to be suffering a good deal from bronchitis. He wished me to look at his legs and feet, but I declined to do so as I was not paying a professional visit. He threw the clothes off the lower part of the bed, and his thighs appeared to be dropsical. His legs below the knees were bandaged, and I could not see their condition. I fancy there was water running away from his legs. I am speaking from only a casual observation. Captain Cain seemed anxious about himself, and asked me if I thought he would suffer more pain. I said I did not think so. He wished me to feel his pulse, and I did so. It struck me that he had a fairly good pulse for a man who was in his condition. I heard of his death the following night, and was rather surprised, judging from what I had seen of him the day before. I know Mrs Hall, the wife of the prisoner. I assisted Dr Macintyre to analyse some ice water on Sunday, 15th August. We analysed it at Watkins' dispensary, after 3 o'clock. We tested it for antimony, and discovered a large quantity in it. We also analysed some urine and vomit on the 13th of August, and found antimony in both. The result was the same in analyses made subsequently. I know that ice was ordered for Mrs Hall, to be given to her in small pieces.

Cross-examined by Mr Chapman: When I saw Captain Cain on the afternoon of the 28th January, he talked a good deal in a disjointed manner. The talk was long and rather distressing. From the character of the cough I should think he had bronchitis. I was in the room for about 10 minutes, I think. I felt Captain Cain's pulse just to comply with his request. He was in a very bad condition, and I knew he had senile mortification of the feet and so on. He was very dropsical. The dropsy might be due to kidney disease, and whatever the source of the dropsy was, it was some pretty well advanced disease. Senile gangrene may be a symptom of, or a sequel to diabetes. Since these proceedings I have looked into the subject of antimonial poisoning. Except as a student I had previously had nothing to do with it. I am not an expert in the subject. From my reading, I should say one man may, under certain conditions, take a larger dose of antimony than another. Persons suffering from certain diseases may take antimony with impunity. The subject of the effects of antimony has not attracted much attention in New Zealand until recently. A medical man I should think could express an opinion with a fair degree of certainty as to the effect of a given dose upon a healthy man. As a general rule, you would find similar symptoms in different persons, but there are exceptions. I have read of a very large dose having been taken, and aid having to be brought in to produce vomiting. In a great many cases, in which the form of the disease is given, I think I could express a positive opinion as to the effect of antimony.

His Honor: It is the case, is it not, that in cases of inflammatory diseases the system can tolerate a greater amount of antimony than under other conditions?—Yes; in acute inflammatory diseases.

Is it the case that in diseases of an exactly contrary kind the converse proposition applies, and that the system would tolerate a much less quantity than under ordinary circumstances?—Decidedy.

What kind of disease was Cain's?—It was one of great weakness.

The converse of an inflammatory disease?—Yes; it was attended with marked depression.

If antimony is administered in small doses to a person who is in the habit of vomiting—who is suffering from a complaint of which vomiting is a symptom—would not the probability be that a great portion of the antimony would be rejected?—If the antimony were given in very minute doses.

Yes; assuming it was given in minute doses?—I should not like to say; I could not answer that question.

Mr Haggitt: Would not the rejection of the antimony depend upon how soon the attack of vomiting followed the administration of the dose?—Naturally it would.

If the fit of vomiting did not come on, we will say, for some considerable interval after the dose of antimony had been administered, what would become of the antimony?—It would remain in the system.

Suppose Captain Cain had been suffering from kidney disease and dropsy, what would be the effect of administering to him small doses of antimony?—I should think it would reduce his vitality still more.

And suppose that in addition to dropsy and kidney disease there was also an affection of the heart, what would be the effect then?—I should think that it would be disastrous—that it would tend to a fatal result.

Mr Chapman: You speak, Dr Drew, with reference to the condition in which you saw Cain on the 28th of January?—Yes.

That is your opinion as a medical man, based on the condition in which you then saw him?—I saw him simply as a casual observer.

And all that you can say is that with this data before you, you give the best opinion you can form under the circumstances?—I knew that Captain Cain had suffered from mortification of the toe and that he had recovered from it, and I knew he was suffering from bronchitis; that was apparent to anybody.

What you have said in reference to these questions is the best opinion you can form with reference to your knowledge and observations of the case?—Yes.

But you do give it as an opinion—you do not speak with absolute certainty as to its necessarily accelerating a man's death, for example? That is simply given as an opinion?—That is the opinion I hold. I certainly think that if antimony were given to a man in that condition it would accelerate his death.

You do not treat it as a matter of certainty. You give the best opinion you can form, which you say is the opinion you hold?—I think it is the opinion of every medical man.

Again, doctor, you put it in the form of an opinion. Is not that so?—Well, I hold a very strong opinion about it.

Yes, but it is an opinion, is it not?—Yes. I have-never had any practical experience beyond this; but from what I have read, and from what I saw and knew of the man's condition, I certainly consider it would accelerate his death.

But that is as far as you will go?—Yes; I hold a very strong opinion upon it.

Hannah Ellison, nurse, residing at Timaru, said: I nursed Mrs Hall from her confinement in June until a month ago, when I left her. She was confined on the 16th June, and took very sick on the third night after her confinement. This sickness continued to the 15th August, off and on. Sometimes she was a couple of days without being sick. She was sick both by day and night. Prisoner was very attentive to her, and used occasionally to give her food and drink. Mrs Hall was very ill on 15th August. She was taking nothing to eat at that time, but only ice and a le ice water to moisten her lips, and I had to give her injections every three hours of brandy, pancreatine, and arrowroot. She was taking nothing by the mouth but ice and ice water. The ice was put on a piece of muslin over a cup, and I poured a little of the ice water from the cup into a wineglass to moisten [ber lips. Other ice broken up was kept on a handkerchief stretched over a jug, and I had filled a colander with ice and put it in the smoking-room adjoining the bedroom so as to be handy for use. The bulk of the ice was kept in the bathroom. The ice that I put on the muslin over the cup on the Saturday night (August 14) I took from the colander. Hall came into Mrs Hall's sick room at about 9 o'clock on Sunday morning, and I left the room when he came in, and stayed away as nearly as I can recollect about half-an-hour. When I returned there was no one in the room but Mrs Hall herself in bed. She looked very ill, and told me that Mr Hall had given her some ice water.

His Honor: I do not think that is evidence.

Witness: She said it had made her feel very sick. She was very sick very soon after I came into the room. In consequence of what Mrs Hall told me I tasted the ice water that was in the cup. It tasted bitter and made me sick. I took about a teaspoonful as nearly as I can guess. I was sick a day and a night some time before that; I do not remember what I had taken. I am not subject to sickness. After tasting the ice water I took the cup containing it, and was going to take it out of the room when Mrs Hall called me back. I then poured part of the water into a clean cup I had in another part of the room on the washstand, and put the first cup back in its place on the dressing table near the bed. I then took the cup I had poured some of the water into out of the room, poured its contents into a little bottle, and put it in my pocket. I then went back into the bedroom, and about five minutes afterwards Mr Hall came in. Mrs Hall asked him to taste the ice water, as it was very nasty, and she complained of being very sick. Hall put it to his lips and said he could not understand it; he must have made a mistake and have poured some of the water out of the jug. Miss Houston came into the room while the conversation was going on, and she said

"If it's nasty you shan't have it," and took the cup and its contents out of the room and brought it back emptied, with clean muslin and more ice on it. I kept the bottle into which I had poured the ice water in my pocket until the doctor came—between 1 and 2 o'clock the same day, and I gave it to him. He took it away with him. Mr Hall used to give me the brandy for the injection. He gave me some that same Sunday. I had some in a bottle in the room, and he gave me some more in a brandy bottle about 6 or 7 o'clock in the evening. The bottle, which was a large one, was not nearly half full. I put it on the chest of drawers in the bedroom, and did not use any of it. Something happened before 9 o'clock (the time for using it) which prevented me. One of the gentlemen called out from the dining room that evening for whisky, saying that Mr Hall was fainting, and I said I had no whisky, but gave the bottle of brandy to Constable Egan. I did not get it back again; the police took it away that night. I after 'this gave everything that passed from Mrs Hall to Dr Macintyre. The police took away the jug containing the ice water; I gave it to Inspector Broham just as it was, with the handkerchief over it, and the water that had trickled through the handkerchief. After the 15th August Mrs Hall's sickness did not continue. The prisoner had no opportunity of attending upon her after that date.

This witness was not cross-examined.

Thomas Broham, inspector of police at Timaru, said: I arrested the prisoner on Sunday, August 15, at about half-past 8 o'clock. Detective Kirby was with me and Constables Egan and Strickland. Prisoner was coming out of the dining room door when I saw him first. He turned back into the dining room and we went in after. Miss Houston was coming out of the smoking room, and I beckoned her to come into the dining room, which she did. I told them I arrested them both on a charge of attempting to poison Mrs Hall by the administration of antimony. Both were very much astonished, and Miss Houston said, "Antimony! Why, that is what you use for your photography." Hall turned to her and said, "Be quiet, you have nothing to do with this." He then said, "What shall I say? I suppose a man ought to be very careful what he says with a charge like this made against him." I said, "You can say anything you please, or nothing at all if you think fit." He then said, "I have used antimony for a long time. I bought tartar emetic at Gunn and Eichbaum's to use with some other things to make into cigarettes for my asthma. You know I suffer from asthma." He then said, "Whatever I did in this matter I did alone. There was no second person concerned in it." He repeated this twice. From the time I went into the room I kept my eyes on Hall's hands. I saw him put them partly into his trousers pockets. I said, "Take your hands out, please; don't move them." Afterwards he made another motion to put them into his pockets, and I said the same thing to him. He began to get very weak, and looked for a nip of brandy, and I sent Constable Egan out to get him some. About this time I told him we would have to search him, and

Kirby and myself went up to do so. He then again asked for brandy, and I thought he seemed very faint, and sent Kirby out of the room to get some as Constable Egan had not returned. Hall had shifted his position, and stood opposite the fire, and directly Kirby left the room he made a sudden movement towards the fire and put his hands into his pockets. I told him to take them out, and he did not do so, and I then siezed his wrists. There was a bright fire burning. We had a struggle. Just then Miss Houston raised a cry, and ran between us, and did all in her power to separate us. We were leaning over the fender, about a foot from the fire, and Hall was making his best exertions, I thought, to throw something into the fire. He did succeed in getting a cork out of his pocket, and I saw it drop on the hearthrug. I called out for Detective Kirby, and as I heard his footsteps approaching, Miss Houston ceased her efforts and stood beside us. I said to Kirby, "He is trying to throw something into the fire," and I held his hands while Kirby searched him, taking out of the right-hand trousers pocket, I think, a small phial containing some fluid and crystal. It had no cork in it. I also saw taken from his pocket a small packet marked "Tartar emetic." The pocket when turned inside out was quite wet. I saw Kirby take a small particle of white powder from the carpet, and also pick up the cork, which fitted the phial. After this Constable Egan brought in a bottle with brandy in it. I saw it looked cloudy, and said to Hall, "There is something wrong with this brandy." He said, "No, it is all right." I said, "You see it is cloudy and dirty looking." He said, "Oh, it is all right at any rate." I am not sure if he or I was pouring some out, but Hall raised the glass to his lips and I stopped him. We then went and searched his bedroom upstairs. On a table I saw a book marked "Taylor on Poisons." Hall reached it before me and said, "I suppose this also will tell against me." I also found in the bedroom some tartar emetic and a bottle of colchicum wine.

Mr Haggit: Anything else?

Witness (after a lengthy pause): Yes. I got a packet of the ordinary shop cigarettes used by people suffering from asthma.

Mr Haggitt asked that these should be produced, and the box containing the exhibits was opened in court.

Witness: We found no home-made cigarettes. All these things were sent to Professor Black for analysis.

To Mr Chapman: It did not come to my notice that a bottle of atropia afterwards came from Hall's office. Kirby gave me a bottle about a month ago which he said he got from Ross. It was labelled "Eye-drops," and is at my office at Timaru now. This was not mentioned at any previous inquiry. I think it was found since the committal. The chemist's name upon the bottle was Eichbaum.

To Mr Haggitt: I searched a drawer in a safe in Hall's office on August 25. I found two policies for insurance for £3000 each. The keys of the safe were found on Hall when arrested.

Austin Kirby, detective at Timaru said: I was present with Inspector Broham when Hall was arrested. Mrs Ellison handed to Constable Egan in my presence a bottle of brandy. I handed it to Inspector Broham, who poured some into a glass. I received this bottle back from him the same evening with a number of other things—all that he got in the house. I kept possession of these till the following morning, when I handed them over to Inspector Brodie, and they were examined in the presence of Dr Macintyre, Constable Daly, and myself. A portion of the contents were sealed up in bottles and given into Constable Daly's charge. I have possession of all the articles in this case, which I received from Dr Ogston at Christchurch on 9th October. His seal is on the box.

To Mr Chapman: I gave Inspector Broham some time ago a small bottle I received from Mr Ross. It contained a light liquid and was a little more than half full. It was, I think, about six weeks after Hall's arrest.

To Mr White: I think it was since his committal.

John Daly, constable at Timaru, said: On August 16 I received some things from Inspector Broham which I packed in a box and took to Dunedin, where I handed them over to Professor Black.

Eugene Egan, constable at Timaru, said: I was present at Hall's arrest on 15th August, and received a bottle containing brandy from Mrs Ellison. I took it into the dining room and poured a portion into a glass. Mr Broham said it had a peculiar colour, and he did not like to give it to Hall to drink. Mr Broham took the bottle.

John William Webb, undertaker, Timaru, said: I knew the late Captain Cain very well and conducted his funeral arrangements. It was at the end of December or beginning of January, I think.

Mr White: Think again.

Witness: I have no doubt. That is when I think it was. I was present at the exhumation.

His Honor: The date of the funeral is important, because it may be a question whether the right body was dug up.

Mr White: We will show it, your Honor.

Witness: I recognised the body as that of Captain Cain. The date of the exhumation was September 27 last, I believe. The coffin was taken out of the same plot that we put it in. We took it from the cemetery to the morgue. Dr Ogston and Dr Hogg were there, and when they had finished, by their orders we closed the coffin again. Drake is the name of the sexton I saw bury the body.

This witness was not cross-examined.

Edward Drake, sexton at the Timaru cemetery, said: I received Captain Cain's coffin from the last witness for burial on 31st January 1886. I afterwards saw it exhumed on 27th September, and taken to the Timaru Hospital, where a post mortem was made by Dr Ogston and Dr Hogg.

Arthur Steadman (recalled) said: The document produced is a mortgage handed me by the prisoner as part security for the overdraft. It was not to be registered at Hall's wish without notice to him. There was a previous mortgage of £4000. In my opinion it became necessary to register it afterwards, and I had it registered. In the interval Hall and Meason had given another mortgage (certified copy produced) over the land for £3500, and ours became a third instead of a second mortgage.

To Mr Chapman: In December and January I was putting no pressure on Hall and Meason. They stood in good credit in my opinion.

Wm. Selig (apprentice to Mr Watkins, chemist, Timaru) deposed: I went into Mr Watkins' employment in October 1882, and have been there ever since. I have made up Captain Cain's cough mixture from Dr Macintyre's prescription. The cough mixture was supplied for the first time on the 24th of December. The entry in the prescription book is in my handwriting, but I cannot swear from that circumstance that I dispensed the prescription. The entry on 13th January is also in my handwriting.

W. H. Willway was recalled, and having examined the books, stated as the result of his examination that Captain Cain had between the 24th December and 28th January 10 bottles of cough mixture prescribed by Dr Macintyre and one other bottle of cough mixture.

Wm. Selig (examination resumed) said: The entry on the 24th of December indicates chlorodyne mixture prescribed by Dr Macintyre. These mixtures were kept made up for him in stock, and we filled a bottle out of the stock as he ordered it. There is an entry on January 13 in my handwriting, "Cough mixture 7144, R.," and on the 14th two similar entries. One is in my handwriting, and one in Mr Stewart's. There is also an entry in my handwriting, "Cough mixture." If it referred to a prescription. I should think a number would be there, and there is no number there. We supplied things to Captain Cain's household that were charged to Captain Cain. The mixture may have been for someone else. We do not know for whose use they are. Is any member of Captain Cain's household bought things they were charged to Captain Cain. On the 23rd, 26th, and 28th of January there are entries of the prescription cough mixture, in my handwriting. The mixture was put into 6oz bottles. The direction on the bottle was, "A dessertspoonful in a little water when pain or cough is troublesome." There were 24 dessertspoonfuls in a bottle.

To Mr Chapman: What was supplied to Captain Cain's household was charged to Captain Cain. I do not know of any purchases for cash having been made for Captain Cain, but there may have been such purchases. There is an entry "Cough mixture" on the 1st December 1884. That was a large bottle Watkins' pectoral, 2s 6d. On 13th November 1885 1oz of strychnine was purchased on Captain Cain's account. I should say about half a dozen different medicines for various purposes are made up and kept in stock for Dr Mac'ntyre. I cannot say if other doctors have prescriptions made up and kept in stock at the other chemists, but we keep no prescriptions in stock for them.

To Mr Haggitt: We have these prescription made up and kept in stock for our own convenience.

Roderick Fraser Stewart, recalled, said: There is an entry in the day book in my handwriting on December 28, 1885, for half a yard of waterproof sheeting and a mixture. The latter is the cough mixture that Dr Macintyre generally prescribes and that we keep in stock. It consists of compound tincture of camphor, chlorodyne, syrup of squills, spirits of nitre, and an infusion of senega. I am able to say from this entry that I supplied the mixture on this date. On 18th January I supplied the same mixture for Captain Cain. I cannot say to whom the strychnine that is entered for Captain Cain on 13th November was given. I could not tell how many made-up medicines prescribed by Dr Macintyre were kept in stock; possibly half-a-dozen—not so many as a dozen.

It being now 5.20 p.m. the adjournment was taken.

Mr Haggitt asked that a number of the witnesses who had been examined should be discharged, as it was a great expense to the country to keep them here.

His Honor allowed a number of the less important witnesses to go.

The court then rose.

Richard Bowen Hogg, deposed: I am a duly qualified medical practitioner, residing and practising at Timaru. I knew the late Captain Cain, and had attended him professionally. Between May and July 1885 I was watching the progress of an affection of one of his eyes. Dr Ferguson was treating him, and I was watching the case for Dr Ferguson. Captain Cain died on the 20th of January 1886. I attended the funeral and saw him buried. I afterwards saw his body exhumed on the night of 27th of September. The coffin was fairly well preserved. The body was taken to the post mortem room of the Timaru hospital. Dr Ogston held the post mortem and I assisted him. I saw the lid removed from the coffin. Considering the length of time the body had been in the ground it was fairly well preserved. I knew Captain Cain very well, and thought I could discern his features. The face was swollen and the hair loose and could be removed by gently pulling. The skin of the face presented a brownish appearance, and the rest of the body had a clayish colour. The backs of the hands and feet were wrinkled and of a blackish colour. The right little toe was missing and the left little toe was hanging by a piece of skin. On cutting the chest and belly the skin and underlying tissues had undergone a change. The heartbag had no fluid in it and the heart itself appeared to be enlarged. The ventricle of the heart seemed dilated and the wall was rather thin. The valve between the ventricle and the auricle was thickened and rigid at its attachment to the wall, but the margins of the valve seemed to be free. The valves of the aorta were also rigid, and had lost their elasticity; they did not close perfectly. The aorta was converted into a bony canal. In young people it is pliable, but in all men of advanced age there is degenerative change of various degrees, but not to that extent. The heart itself was rather foxy. In the left ventricle there was a little fluid blood. The lungs were of a dark red colour of congested appearance, but elastic and fairly bulky. In the lateral cavities of the chest there was a bloody fluid equal to about from three to four pints. The stomach and intestines looked well preserved; externally they presented a sort of greyish pink appearance. There was a little fluid in the abdominal cavity—from an ounce to an ounce and a-half. The bowels appeared to be empty. On opening the stomach there was a greyish mucous covering the surface, which was also present to some extent in the intestines adjoining the stomach. The wall of the stomach seemed rather thin. In the bladder there was about 4oz of urine. The liver was smooth on the surface, presenting a greyish brown colour, and one section appeared to be fairly healthy. The kidneys, so far as one could tell after that lapse of time, appeared to be healthy, as well as the spleen. I consider the internal parts of the body were well preserved, and remarked that at the time. Captain Cain had been buried about eight months. After so long a lapse of time it is difficult to give an opinion as to whether or not the liver and kidneys had been diseased. Portions of the viscera were removed. The bladder was emptied, and its contents and the bladder, and fluid from the cavity of the abdomen, and fluid from the cavities of the chest were removed. A portion of the liver, the whole of the spleen and the kidneys were also taken. These were placed in four clean wide-mouthed bottles, which were corked, covered with parchment, and sealed with Dr Ogston's private seal. They remained in his possession until we arrived in Dunedin, and they were then handed over to Professor Black at the University. The seals were then broken and the contents of the bottles analysed. The contents of each bottle were analysed separately. We tested for antimony. We did not test for colchicum, considering that all trace of vegetable poison would be destroyed by that time. Atropia is also a vegetable poison. The tests were confirmatory: antimony was found in each case. Reinsch's test and sulphuretted hydrogen gas, and a test by hydrochloric acid and cloride of potash were also used. These tests were variously applied over and over again, except in one or two instances, in which an error was made in the process, which was corrected afterwards. Professor Black and Dr Ogston made the tests and I performed one analysis myself. (The process of analysis was then described.) Antimony is a metal, and besides being a metal is an irritant poison. I am not aware that metallic antimony is a poison. Tartar emetic is the salt of antimony—antimony in combination with cream of tartar. Tartar emetic is a poison. It might be a poison from two grains upwards.

Mr Haggitt: Is it more likely to be fatal in small doses frequently repeated or in a large dose?

Witness: It is more likely to be poisonous in small doses frequently repeated. A large dose would give rise to vomiting, and it would be all or nearly all thrown off, while in small doses it would be retained and absorbed into the system. Tartarised antimony, especially if in solution, is quickly absorbed into the system. If a person took antimony and was not sick immediately afterwards it would commence to be absorbed into his blood in a few minutes. If absorbed into the blood its action depends on the dose. In a medicinal dose it may act as a sedative upon the brain and heart. It might be administered medicinally to children for croup, bronchitis, and inflammation of the lungs, but in very small doses. Those are the only cases in which it would be used. Years ago it was used in typhus fever, but is it not so used now. A medicinal dose is from 1-16th of a grain to an eighth of a grain to promote perspiration. A slightly larger dose, from ⅛ to ¼ of a grain, would act as a sedative, and a larger dose still as an emetic. In the case of a larger dose still being given, signs of irritation of the intestinal canal would occur, producing vomiting and purging with pain, and great depression of the heart, and if continued, exhaustion and death. I have been speaking of the effect of it on an ordinarily healthy person.

Supposing it to be administered to a person in a generally enfeebled state of health, suffering from general debility, with kidney disease, constipation, and dropsy, what would be the effect? Very injurious.

How would it act in such a case as that?—By increasing the debility and hastening the result of the disease.

When a person is in a condition such as that I have mentioned, does he require stimulants and nourishing?—He may require stimulants. Of course it depends upon the case. I cannot speak generally.

Are depressants good for him, then, under any circumstances?—I should say not.

Tartar emetic, I understand you to say, administered in small doses, acts as a depressant?—Yes.

And the result of administering depressants to a person in that state is what?—Injurious; and if continued long enough fatal.

Suppose antimony to be administered in large doses to a person in such a state?—It would have a very depressing effect.

And supposing that continued large doses were given, what would be the effect?—It would be still more depressive.

If these doses were continued, what would be the effect of them?—They would be fatal.

Witness (continued): If antimony is administered and taken into the blood it gives rise to irritation of the intestinal canal, epecially vomiting and purging, great weakness of the heart, very great depression; and if the administration was persisted in it would produce death from exhaustion.

Mr Haggitt: Supposing in any patient you found nausea, continued vomiting, diarrhœa followed by constipation, then diarrhœa again depression, and loss of strength, would they indicate anything to you?—They would indicate irritation, probably by poison. It depends upon whether the patient was in a good state of health or whether he was suffering from a long illness. In a person previously healthy, what would they indicate?—If these symptoms suddenly arose, I should looked for an irritant. Of course it might be English cholera. It would depend on the season of the year and where you were. It might be a number of other things, I suppose, too?—Yes.

Well, if a person had shown such symptoms in his life and dies, and on *post mortem* analysis of the internal organs of his body you discovered the presence of antimony, what would that indicate?—It would indicate that the antimony had been the cause of those symptoms. You are saying a healthy person?

Suppose now, then, the case of a person who had been suffering from old age and debility, and the diseases Dr Macintyre spoke of, and you discovered antimony in the body, what would that indicate to you?—That it might be the cause of the symptoms described by Dr Macintyre. Does it indicate anything else?—Vomiting and diarrhœa are occasionally symptoms of disease of the kidneys, but much more frequently of irritant poisoning, and if continued they are persistent, whereas in disease they would be intermittent—only occasional.

It being stated by Dr Macintyre that Captain Cain suffered from nausea, vomiting, thirst, depression, increasing weakness, and diarrhœa, and that these symptoms continued the same with increasing weakness down to the time of his death, and knowing that you yourself found antimony in the body after death, what do you conclude?—That they are more consistent with the symptoms of antimonial poisoning.

One more question : Supposing the symptoms to be the same as I last put them to you, although they were even traceable to disease, and you found antimony after death, what would you conclude?—That the antimony had greatly aggravated the disease ; that it had hastened the fatal termination of the disease.

That is, in other words, that antimony administered under such circumstances accelerated death?—Yes.

Cross-examined by Mr Chapman: I have given these last answers as my own inference and from my general knowledge and from reading cases from authorities. Granger Stuart is one of the authorities I referred to. He is an authority on kidney diseases ; not on antimonial poisoning. Woodman and Tidy I take as an authority on antimonial poisoning. It is a comparatively recent work, and I recognise it as a standard authority. Another authority is Taylor, an old standard work. I do not recollect other authorities just now, but I may have read smaller works. I was familiar before last winter with the subject that antimony would accelerate every exhausting disease that I can think of just now. Antimony would accelerate every disease that was attended with general debility and weakness of

the heart's action. That is my opinion. I do not dogmatise on the subject, but express an opinion from my general knowledge and my reading of certain works. Prior to last reading I had no experience of such a case as it, but I had experience of the physiological results of antimony administered in disease. I have had occasion to stop it in cases I have treated. I have found it produce too much depression. I have had occasion to stop it in cases of pneumonia, where diarrhœa has come on, because I considered I had gone far enough. I have not observed the over-action of antimony in my patients. I seldom prescribe it ; but I have prescribed it within the last six months, and with good results. That was in a case of inflammation of the lungs. Antimony under such circumstances as were described by Mr Haggitt would, in my opinion, accelerate death.

Mr Chapman : That is only given as an opinion ?—In the case of an old man 70 years of age, with infirmity of the heart, disease of the kidneys, and dropsy—allowing that he was not subject to that condition of system which is called idiosyncrasy — I most unhesitatingly affirm that antimony in small doses would accelerate death.

You have in your last answer put out of count one element ?—The element of idiosyncrasy.

That is individual peculiarity ?—Yes.

Witness continued : The opinion I have just given is founded apart from that. There might be idiosyncrasy which would affect the result. I have not given that answer with reference to any particular quantity of the dose and without reference to the frequency of the dose. My opinion is that a single dose in a case of that kind of extreme debility would increase depression and accelerate death. I should be very sorry to give in such a case one dose of two grains or to give repeatedly much smaller doses. From one to two grains is spoken of in the authorities as an emetic dose. I have never administered it as an emetic. It is very little used as an emetic now. The medical profession abandoned its use as an emetic because it was so slow in its action. Now and then you will get a case where you will not get an emetic effect, but such cases are rare, and I should think are cases of fever.

Mr Chapman : Can you refer me to any authority for saying that diarrhœa and vomiting are occasional if disease of the kidneys is present, and that in irritant poisoning,.if continued, they are persistent ? What is your authority for saying that in disease they are intermittent ? —Granger Stuart is my authority, I think, for saying that they are often intermittent.

And for the other : their continuousness in irritant poisoning ?—Up to a certain point they would be intermittent.

We will take one question at a time. You have given us your authority for one-half of your proposition ; I should like the authority for the other ?—I fancy Taylor.

Your answer was that in disease they may be intermittent ?—Yes.

We may also take it, I suppose, that in disease they may be continuous?—I should not like to say they might not be.

When you say that in irritant poisoning they would be continuous, do you mean that, or do you mean that they would be persistent in irritant poisoning if the application of the poison was continuous?—You are talking about very different states of the system. May I explain to you that in typhus fever——

There was no talk about typhus fever when these answers were given to Mr Haggitt. What he was wishing to get at was whether the symptoms observed were more probably attributable to disease or to poisoning. You then gave it as your idea that vomiting and diarrhœa are occasional in disease of the kidneys, but you said that in irritant poisoning they are persistent. Does not tha: depend upon the persistency of the poisoning?—Yes, persistent administration—and I wish to guard myself here. I admitted that large doses have been administered and that four or five doses might not have an emetic effect, but that would be in cases of typhus; and in cases where there is a high temperature there is no secretion of the gastric juice, but if you take a non-febrile disease in an old man——

Let us keep to one thing at a time. I was asking you, not with reference to any answers you have given me, but with reference to answers to questions by Mr Haggitt. I think that you have now answered that the persistence of vomiting produced by irritant poisoning would be dependent upon the continuous administration of the poison?—Yes, in small doses.

His Honor : That is to say, if the doses were dropped off for a day or two the symptoms of vomiting would disappear?—I think they would.

Mr Chapman : Would not symptoms of vomiting disappear if the doses were dropped for a day or two?—The patient might suffer from nausea. It might not abruptly cease with the administration of poison, but I should not expect it to last very long.

Witness continued: I know that antimony is very often beneficial in chest affections, in small doses, but you have to consider the condition of the patient. When I was at the Timaru hospital I prescribed it in small doses occasionally. I think antimony is used in some patent medicine, and that the compound syrup of squills is in the American Pharmacopœia.

Mr Chapman : Can you, after hearing the symptoms described by Dr Macintyre, say what Captain Cain was suffering from ?

Witness : Kidney disease of some sort.

But what kind of kidney disease ?—I happened to know something about Captain Cain. I know he had heart disease. I could not form an idea as to what the nature of the kidney disease was from merely seeing the patient. I could not tell without analysing the urine. That is essential in diagnosing to ascertain the particular form of kidney disease. If I had had a patient of the kind I should probably have made the examination. I should certainly have made it.

Had the case been in your hands you might have examined the urine after death ?—A doctor is generally supposed to have made up his mind, if possible, as to the nature of the illness before death. You could get urine after death to examine, if there was any in the bladder. You heard Dr Macintyre's description of the symptoms : was there anything in them to suggest Bright's disease?—I cannot answer that question. The vomiting is perhaps suggestive of it.

Is the diarrhœa suggestive of it ?—There might be diarrhœa in Bright's disease.

Is there thirst ?—I do not know that that is a marked symptom. It depends whether there would be much drain from the system. I am not aware that thirst is a leading characteristic of Bright's disease. I have had a medical man's ordinary experience of that disease. I have not marked thirst as a symptom.

Is it inconsistent with Bright's disease ?—I should not like to say that. It depends, as I said, upon the drain from the system. Bright's disease is a very wasting and weakening one.

What is its leading feature?—General debility. What is found in Bright's disease is albumen in the urine. You do not always get it. You may have other things. I would not conclude a man had Bright's disease only because I found albumen in the urine.

But would it not be the first thing you looked for?—Yes, it would. I recognise Professor Granger Stuart as a special authority on kidney disease.

If you found him making special reference to thirst as a symptom, would you consider that he attached special importance to it ?—I should.

Mr Chapman then read a passage from the work in question in which albumen was mentioned.

Witness : Will you tell me what form of Bright's disease that was?

Does your answer to my question as to thirst depend upon the form of Bright's disease?—Witness (after a pause) : I don't know that it does.

Then what makes you ask me the particular form of the disease in the case I read ? I should like to know. Why did you ask me the question ? Because in some forms of Bright's disease there is more copious excretion of urine than others. That would have something to do with the question of thirst.

Then in some cases you would expect thirst to be a feature ? It might be. I do not suppose Professor Stuart would have mentioned thirst unless he attached some importance to it. Diminished power of sight is also a feature of some forms of Bright's disease. I have been reading up this subject for some days to assist me in answering questions here. I have also been reading up the subject of antimonial poisoning.

And a good many of your replies are the result of this reading?—The result of refreshing my memory.

By reading books you had read before ?—No; not the same book. I daresay I have also talked upon the subject with Dr Drew. Kidney disease has been the subject of conversation in many ways. I have discussed other features of the case with Dr Batchelor—no doubt to get enlightenment and see if our opinions agreed. I have talked with Dr Ogston about the analysis and the symptoms of Cain's disease, also with Dr Brown. Lately?—Since I have come down here—on Thursday week. Yesterday was the most recent occasion with Dr Brown. I have discussed my evidence to-day with Dr Brown.

Then you have, so to speak, built up your recollections upon your former studies and recent reading and conversation with other gentlemen?—Yes.

You spoke some time ago about James' powder. You do not use that?—No. I daresay it has been used in Bright's disease by other medical men—in an acute form of the disease, not in a chronic case. I recognise Sir William Roberts as an authority. I have had his book for some time.

You say, then, that the use of James' powder does not apply to chronic cases and is limited to acute forms of the disease?—I think so. I should not think anyone would prescribe it in chronic Bright's disease.

Do you think Sir William Roberts would prescribe and recommend it?—He might probably do so in an acute attack on a chronic form of the disease.

Mr Chapman (showing witness a chapter in Sir William Roberts' work on chronic Bright's disease): Do you see any reference to an acute access there?—Witness: No; I do not.

Suppose you found albumen in the urine of a patient, would you not attribute it to Bright's disease?—Not necessarily. It might be due to a cardiac disease giving rise to congestion of the kidneys. I should not attribute the symptoms to Bright's disease without making a further examination. It might be my first inclination to do so.

Do you recognise the new classification of Bright's disease spoken of by Dr Macintyre?—Bright himself looked upon all diseases of the kidneys as Bright's disease. So did some writers subsequent to Bright, down to the date, I suppose, when the microscope came into use some 25 years ago.

Then do you suppose Dr Macintyre belonged to the anti-microscopical period until he furbished himself up before appearing in the lower court?—I do not say that. I became a medical man in 1870. My education was based upon what Dr Macintyre called the new classification.

With reference to squills, ammonia, and senega, are they irritants to the stomach?—In large doses they are and might produce sickness. Opium might produce vomiting. In some cases squills and senega might act as irritants to the bowels.

Did you give Mr Haggitt a minute and detailed description of all you did at the post mortem?—I think I did. I assisted in putting the contents into the bottles. Dr Ogston actually did all the cutting and lifting out of the pieces, tying, &c. Dr Macintyre, the steward of the hospital, and Dr Drew were present; also the undertaker and sexton, and I fancy Mr Perry. We began the post mortem at about half-past 10 at night, and finished be-

tween 12 and 1 o'clock. My part was witnessing and assisting Dr Ogston. I think I have described every part of the body we opened. We did not open the skull at all, or the spinal column. Mr White, the Crown solicitor at Timaru, first asked me to take part in this proceeding, and I declined. Dr Macintyre asked me again, because there was no one else left to assist, and then I consented. I think Mr White mentioned that Dr Ogston was coming. He said I was to assist him in making the examination of the body. Dr Macintyre urged me to assist because he thought Dr Ogston would like to have someone to assist him.

What was it led you to select all those particular parts of the body?—I did not select them; it was Dr Ogston. I left it entirely in his hands. I judged that he selected these particular parts to look for poison. In my opinion they seemed the most suitable parts to select, in order to get the alimentary canal and those portions of the viscera I have mentioned. Mineral irritants are deposited in those particular organs.

Then you did not think it was necessary that Dr Ogston should trouble himself about anything but mineral irritants?—Dr Ogston is a medical jurist.

But you exercised your reason. Do you know nothing about medical jurisprudence?—Oh, yes; I did not think it necessary to recommend his taking anything else, because I thought he had sufficient for a search for mineral irritants. We found a large quantity of fluid in the lung cavities. I thought this might be an exudation of blood from the base of the lungs, which occurred very likely just before death, or even immediately after. We did not examine the smaller vessels. You would infer from the condition of the large vessels that there would be disease of the smaller ones.

In Cain's case, what would you expect to result if, say, he had too much champagne given him—twice as much as the doctor intended?—That depends——

What does it depend on?—Well, champagne might be given to relieve sickness.

But suppose twice, or four times as much as the doctor intended was given in 24 hours, would that relieve sickness?—It all depends on the condition of the patient. I do not think it would produce vomiting in a case like Captain Cain's.

No excess of champagne?—An excess might. It might also produce purging. In conducting the post mortem we found the left ventricle of the heart somewhat dilated. This I ascribed to gurgitation of blood from the aorta.

Would it be a symptom of Bright's disease?—No.

Not in any form?—I will not say that.

In what form?—Well, it would have to be in a contracted form.

What you saw in the left ventricle, then, is characteristic of a form of Bright's disease?—Well, there was no hypertrophe or thickening of the wall of the ventricle. Disease of the aorta or arteries is often an accompaniment of Bright's disease.

Re-examined by Mr Haggitt: There are a great many forms of Bright's disease, and the symptoms vary in nearly every case. By the simplest classification there are three forms. Some medical men, even at the present day, look upon all albumen as indicating a disease of the kidney structure.

Does this in every case produce vomiting?— You may have vomiting in every form. The cause of vomiting is retention of urea. It is the result of uremic poisoning. This is not an accompaniment of every form of kidney disease, In passive kidney disease—conjestion of the kidneys—I would not expect to find uremic poisoning.

What form of kidney disease was Cain suffering from?—I saw nothing during life to show that he was suffering from Bright's disease. After death one could not form a definite idea of the condition of the kidney, so I could not form a conclusion on the subject. Cain had dropsy in the legs, I believe. I did not see him for some time before his death. In Bright's disease you may have dropsy in the ankles, the face, or the hands. Sometimes you have no dropsy in Bright's disease. It generally comes first in the face, about the eyelids and under the eyes. You do not have it in the thighs before it comes in the face.

His Honor: Has uremic poisoning any connection with dropsy? — Witness: Not with dropsy depending upon heart or liver disease.

To Mr Haggitt: I was attending Cain between May and July 1885. He was suffering from disease of the heart then. There was an unnatural murmur over the base of the heart, and I found he had disease of the aortic valves.

Are you aware of any idiosyncrasy in Cain's case which would render antimony innoxious to him?—No, I am not aware of any such idiosyncrasy. The effect of the administration of antimony to a person with such heart disease as Cain's would be very depressing. I know the cough mixture which Dr M'Intyre prescribes. I think I took it once for a cold.

Mr Chapman : Not from Cain's bottles ? Witness : No.

Mr Chapman : From Watkins' tap, I suppose. Witness (to Mr Haggitt): Whether opium produced sickness would depend on the quantity. A fifteenth of a grain to a dose ought not to produce vomiting. In rare cases it might make one sick. Whether squills and ammonia produced irritation of the bowels would also depend upon the quantity. I was asked to assist at the post mortem because I was the only medical man not connected with the case in Timaru.

To Mr Chapman : Captain Cain visited me between May and July three days. Dropsy in Bright's disease is at the beginning confined to the face, the hands, and the ankles.

Invariably ?—Yes, in the face invariably. You may have it in the morning in the face and at night in the ankles. It is usual, but it does not necessarily appear at all. Dropsy and uremia are both characteristics of Bright's disease. It is not easy to diagnose it, though, unless you examine the water. By only seeing the patient you would have a difficulty in diagnosing uremia from apoplexy if he was quite unconscious. There might also be partial insensibility from apoplexy. Also there might be alcoholism. Apart from alcoholism the difficulty would lie between uremia and apoplexy. Either of these conditions may arise from Bright's disease.

William Brown, medical practioner in Dunedin, said: I am a bachelor of medicine, and have been practising for 16 or 17 years.

Mr Haggitt : What would be the effect of tartar emetic administered in such quantities as to cause vomiting to a person suffering from kidney disease and dropsy ?—It would be very dangerous, unless the kidney disease was of a certain nature, when the effect of the remedy would not be very dangerous, but risky. I refer to acute kidney disease.

Suppose there was also something wrong with the heart ?—I should say then that doses large enough to produce sickness and vomiting would be extremely dangerous.

Suppose, in addition, the patient had been suffering from general debility? — It would probably kill him.

Suppose he were suffering from senile gangrene, vomiting, and diarrhœa? — The effect would be to kill him unless he vomited a portion of it up. Still the postration might cause death even if he did so.

Mr Chapman (cross-examining): Have you given the subject of antimony special study?— Not very, except during the last few days, when I have refreshed my memory. I am a partner of Dr Ogston's, and have discussed it in a general way with him since the case became a matter of notoriety.

Francis Ogston, doctor of medicine of Aberdeen University, and lecturer on medical jurisprudence at the Otago University, said : I have made poisons a subject of special study at Prague. I attended a course of lectures from the public toxicologist of Bohemia, and passed an examination in analysis, and am therefore competent to practise as an analyst in Germany. I was for 10 years licensed lecturer on toxicology at Aberdeen, and was as an expert employed for the Crown in all medico-legal cases in Aberdeen. I was police surgeon for years. My father was a toxicologist, and I edited a book on poisons written by him. I was present when the body of Captain Cain was disinterred, and I performed the post mortem, in a shed belonging to the Timaru Hospital, on 27th September last. The first thing was to examine and identify the coffin. The grave clothes were then opened and examined by me. I saw no evidence of the body having been meddled with. I examined the toes for purpose of identification, and found the right little toe wanting.

Mr Haggitt: What was the outward appearance of the body?

Witness : It struck me as rather well preserved for the time it had been in the grave. The skin was yellowish-grey or buff colour, like leather. There was not the usual smell of putridity so strong as I expected. I opened the body as far as I thought useful. I omitted the head because in the case of an old body the brain is only a mass of pulpy fluid after that lapse of time. I have made about 500 post mortem examinations—sometimes of old bodies,—and have often opened the head and found I could make nothing of it.

You opened the body, and what was its appearance?—There was plenty of fat beneath the skin, which was converted into a sort of tallowy mass. I opened down the front, exposing the belly and chest. I examined first the chest and found the lungs dark and moderately spongy. I put my hand between the lungs and ribs and turned out one lung and looked at the pleural cavity. In it I found a moderate quantity of red fluid. I then opened the heart bag and found no fluid in it. I opened the heart and found it rather large and heavy, but the walls seemed about a natural thickness, though the lower cavity was somewhat enlarged. The valves contained bony plates. This is not unusual in old people. The main artery of the body was simply converted into a rigid bony tube for the whole length and its second and third divisions. This was very unusual to such an extent.

Mr Haggitt: What did it indicate?—I think it indicated that the man had a wonderful constitution to live as long as he did with that state of the arteries. The valves between the cavity of the heart and the aorta were diseased. The largeness and flabbiness of the heart in connection with the bony aorta indicated disease.

From the extent of this bony tube could you form an idea how long there had been disease of the heart?—It must have existed for some years. I next proceeded to examine the lungs, taking them out in the usual manner, and found a quantity of blood or bloody fluid. They were healthy enough. The liver, spleen, and kidneys were looked at, but the change that had taken place made it impossible to say whether they were diseased or not. All we could say was that they were not much diseased, if at all. The stomach was taken out with part of the beginning of the small bowel, and opened and looked at simply. A piece from the centre of the small bowel and part of the large bowel here and there were opened and looked at. They all contained a coating of greyish slime more or less, but no *fæces.* The urinary bladder was opened and found to contain about four ounces of urine. It was clear, not muddy, flaky, or thick. The cavity of the belly and the glands attached to the bowels were quite healthy. I was running my hand down the whole length of the spinal column and could discover no fracture, either old or new. There was a gall stone in the gall bladder, but that is a very common thing. The quantity of fat in the body indicated to a certain degree good bodily nourishment. It indicated that the food taken had nourished the body, and had not gone away to waste, but that digestion was good. The red fluid in the pleural cavity indicated that he had lain in the grave a good time, and that he had died slowly. The fluid state of the blood in the heart was a little inconsistent with slow death from natural causes, and was a little suspicious. The main object of the *post mortem* was not so much to find the cause of death as to find poison. I took away some of the bloody fluid

and blood glands for the sake of the blood. Then I took away, in the second place, the intestinal trach and the urinary bladder, urine, and the kidneys. The first represent absorption, the second retention, and the third elimination. I put them in new wide-mouthed bottles, which had been carefully washed out with strong acid and distilled water. I corked the bottles, covered them securely, and sealed them. I then kept them in my possession until I delivered them over to Dr Black with the seals unbroken. In all this I was assisted by Dr Hogg, but in every detail of it I did everything myself. I saw Dr Black lock them up in a room. I went home, had some food, and then returned, and we commenced the analysis of the contents of the still unbroken bottles. We made a preliminary analysis of a little of the fluid from each of the bottles. Bottle No. 3 contains stomach and part of small bowel; No. 1, urinary bladder, kidneys, a little fluid, and small intestine; No. 4, parts of large bowel and liver, and spleen; No. 2, bloody fluid from pleural cavities. I or Dr Black, or Dr Hogg made a preliminary analysis that night and found in each antinony. We used three tests—Reinsch's test, the tin test, and the zinc and platinum test. We got the same result by each test. In each case are produced the metal antimony. The next day we confirmed our test by taking larger quantities and destroying the solids and reducing them to fluids. We then submitted the fluids to the three tests mentioned. We also submitted part of them to another test and I found a trifling indication of antimony before the test, which would take 12 hours, was completed. The test was completed by Drs Black and Hogg. The other tests were quite satisfactory, antimony being discovered in each of them. These tests were also confirmed by experiments made with the solution obtained from the last-named test. We repeatedly tested all the chemicals used. The only deposit one could mistake for antimony would be arsenic, and a test that was made by heating a piece of copper with the deposit on it showed that it could not be arsenic. I can swear that the result of the tests was to indicate the presence of antimony in the remains. We brought some of the earth from the grave, tested two pounds of it, and found no antimony in it. We found the body unusually well preserved. Antimony is a preservative. I have nothing to add respecting the analysis.

Mr Haggitt: From the *post mortem* appearances of the body and your finding this antimony, can you form any opinion as to the cause of death?—The death must have been one of exhaustion.

Would antimony cause exhaustion?—Certainly.

You have heard the state of Captain Cain's health read. What would be the effect of tartar emetic administered to a person in his state of health?—It would be highly dangerous.

And supposing tartar emetic had been administered in doses sufficient to cause vomiting, what would have been the result?—It would have increased every symptom of his natural illness.

Witness continued: The effect of antimony upon the human body is depressing, but in a very large dose it acts as an irritant. In small doses it acts partly as an irritant, partly as a depressant, and occasions a large flow of bile, the result of which would be diarrhœa and bilious vomiting. I believe antimony is quickly absorbed into the body, every soluble poison is quickly absorbed. All the poison that is not rejected is not absorbed; probably a good deal of it would be thrown down as an insoluble sulphide into the stomach and bowels. If the patient lives, that may be absorbed, as there are many acids in the bowels which may or may not dissolve it. The most prominent symptom of antimonial poisoning is sickness coming on very shortly after the poison is taken; then you have purging, great exhaustion, and periods of apparent recovery in the morning if the poison is not given during the night. Thirst, as is the case in all irritant poisons, is a prominent symptom, and also griping of the throat.

Mr Haggitt: Taking it as a fact that Captain Cain during the last portion of his illness, say the last fortnight, suffered from nausea, vomiting, diarrhœa, depression, loss of strength, the weakness gradually increasing, and taking in conjunction with that the *post mortem* appearance you observed, and the fact that on analysis antimony was found in the body, what conclusion would you arrive at?—That antimony had a great deal to do with his death.

His Honor: You say, doctor that you found antimony in the intestines and in the urine as well as in the blood?—Yes.

After the antimony goes into the mouth, what is the ordinary course of things; into the stomach first, I suppose?—Yes, first into the stomach; then it is absorbed into the blood, and acts as a poison there. Part of it would remain insoluble in the bowels, part would be absorbed in the blood, and that absorbed part would be eliminated by the urine.

It must be absorbed before it could reach the urine?—Yes.

All these natural processes would come to an end at death?—Yes.

From the fact of antimony having been found in the urine, could you form any inference as to how long before death the antimony must have been administered?—No; not without referring to some books on physiology. It could be found out by giving certain substances and waiting till they come out in the urine.

You could fix a period within which it would happen?—Yes; it must have been within eight or ten hours. Soluble bodies entering into the body would come out into the urine within eight or ten hours at the outside.

Might it not have been administered before that?—It must have been, because a good deal was lying in the bowels, and all that we found in the lower bowel might have been administered days before, and what was in the stomach a few hours before death.

Can you draw any inference from what you found as to the time at which it was administered, the size of the doses in which it was administered, and further, can you draw any inference as to whether what you found in the

body was all that was administered?—We did not find all that was administered, for we knew very well that diarrhœa would carry off a great portion of it, as we found on a former analysis; antimony being effective upon the liver, making a flow of bile, would act as any other purgative, and it might go into the stomach and out of the bowels within six or eight hours. Then if you find antimony in a man's body and before he dies he suffered from diarrhœa, there is a probability that the antimony found in the body was not all the antimony aministered to him?—It would not be all the antimony probably? If antimony was found in a man's body and shortly before his death he had been suffering from diarrhœa, then I should presume the antimony had caused the diarrhœa.

And that the diarrhœa would itself have carried off a good deal of it?—Yes.

Where antimony has been administered for a period, are there any appearances of the intestines that would indicate that it had been so administered?—Yes. If the dose was a sufficiently graded one to be retained for a little time, and yet large enough to act with its full virulence upon the stomach, there would be inflammation; but if there were smaller doses repeated you would have less signs—irritation instead of inflammation.

Did you observe any signs on the bowels, or were they too far decomposed?—They were decomposed pretty much, and as soon as decomposition sets in all redness would disappear; but we had a coating of dirty grey film.

What does that mean?—It means that some inflammation occurred—perhaps chronic, perhaps lasting for some time. And in that film we found antimony. Then we had a negative indication; we had no signs of any inflammatory disease, because that would cause either ulceration in the bowels themselves or enlargement of the mesenteric glands.

Perhaps you will be good enough, before tomorrow if you can, to look up the subject I was referring to and ascertain, if possible, how long antimony might have been administered?—Yes.

Can you draw any inference as to the doses in which it had been administered? I ask that question because I see that in cases of poisoning by arsenic doctors profess to be able to do so.—There are so many modes of rejection that any inference as to quantities is vitiated. The poison we found lying in the mucous of the bowels was insoluble and unabsorbed, and was not the stuff that actually poisoned him.

Tartar emetic is a poison and antimony is a metal, is it not?—Yes.

What you found in the body was metal antimony, I suppose?—No. We found some form of antimony, but not the metal antimony, in the bowels; probably it was sulphide of antimony.

The antimony must have been administered during life?—Yes.

Can you say it was administered in the form of tartar emetic?—No; that is impossible.

It must have been administered in a soluble form?—Yes. If you asked for antimony you would probably get tartar emetic.

To Mr Haggitt: Our tests bring it back to the metal antimony. I assisted Dr Black in performing some analysis previously in connection with another case with which the prisoner was concerned. On September 12 I analysed certain things brought from Dr Macintyre's laboratory by Dr Black, which were sealed by my seal. I sealed and labelled everything I took over so as to identify it again. The analysis all showed antimony distinctly. Another analysis on the 19th gave similar results. The ice water tested on August 29 in Dr Macintyre's house, at Timaru, must have been saturated with antimony. Colchicum was found in some brandy we tested. We tested some cigarettes in Christchurch, but found no antimony in them. Antimony is not used in making cigarettes. Except you wanted to kill somebody, you would not put antimony in cigarettes. Antimony used in cigarettes could not possibly be of any use in asthma. I have used antimony in medical practice, but it is very little used. We have safer and better means now to secure the same objects it was used for. I analysed a trousers pocket and traced antimony in it. I had a phial said to have been taken from the prisoner's trousers pocket to test. In that phial we found a soluble antimony.

Mr Haggitt said he might ask Dr Ogston a few more questions in the morning.

The court adjourned at 20 minutes past 5 o'clock.

SATURDAY, JANUARY 29.

SIXTH DAY OF THE TRIAL.

Mr Haggitt: Dr Ogston, I understand, has looked up the matter your Honor yesterday requested him to, and is now able to give the information your Honor requires.

Dr Ogston, whose examination was resumed, said : I have looked up so far as I could several authorities, and have the books here. I find several things to go upon as we wished. The first I would refer to is "Carpenter's Physiology," page 159, where he says——

His Honor : Give us the conclusion you have framed from the books?

Witness : Certain substances easily soluble may appear in the urine 12 minutes after being taken if taken after a substantial meal. Another substance—fero-cyanide of potassium—if taken on an empty stomach, has been found in the bladder from one to two and a-half minutes after being taken. Then in a German book which I have here, speaking of arsenic, it says : It is found in urine even after five or six hours. That means as soon as five or six hours. The more soluble compound of arsenic—arsenite of potash—has been found an hour afterwards.

His Honor : I understand the antimony found in the bladder, therefore, may have been taken within a short period of death?

Witness : Yes. I have a last reference here from "Taylor on poisons," with regard to antimony. I may say when speaking of arsenic, the author says, " These remarks apply to antimony." Taylor speaking of poisons, page 30, says "It may be found in the urine passed a few hours afterwards." If your Honor would allow me, I would remark on the great inconvenience I have

been put to in this case by the want of a medical library at the University. I have had to borrow books from my friends. I should like to state that publicly, because of the great inconvenience I have been put to.

His Honor : In time, I hope, our resources will enable us to have a sufficient medical library at the University. It is a question of money.

Mr Chapman : Wool is rising, your Honor.—(Laughter.)

His Honor : It may be detected then, but it does not follow that it was administered within a few hours. Is it not possible that antimony found in the urine may be the elimination of a quantity of antimony administered a very considerable time before?

Witness : Oh, yes.

His Honor : Though it may have been administered a short time before, you cannot say that it was?

Witness : I cannot.

His Honor : The antimony found in the intestines had not been absorbed, I understand?

Witness : That had not been absorbed. In certain conditions of the stomach it is thrown down as an insoluble compound. That would occur in cases where the patient was suffering from wasting disease and not taking food ; in cases where the appetite is destroyed.

His Honor : Could you tell how long before death this antimony so thrown down must have been taken?

Witness : Well, if there were no digestion going on the antimony might remain any time. Antimony is soluble in acids, and there may be no antimony absorbed if there are no acids freed from the stomach. In ordinary cases gastric juice is thrown out to meet any food that is thrown down. That acid acts upon the food and breaks it up, but where digestion is destroyed, or very greatly weakened, there would be no gastric juice thrown out, and consequently the antimony would not be dissolved.

His Honor : I gather from what you say that you really cannot tell when this antimony that was in the intestines was administered ; that it might have been administered the moment before death for all you know?

Witness : Yes, some of it.

His Honor : Or at any time before. You have nothing to guide you as to the period before death when it was administered?

Witness : No, I think not.

His Honor : The antimony that was found in the intestines had not been acted upon by the gastric juice?

Witness : Quite so.

His Honor : Is it possible that when a dose of antimony has been taken part of it may be acted upon by the gastric juices, be absorbed and go into the circulation, and that another part of it might remain in the intestines?

Witness : Oh yes.

His Honor : Is there anything to show the time and the amount of the doses?

Witness : Nothing at all.

His Honor : Could you tell from the examination of the body whether there were any indications of uremic poisoning?

Witness : I saw none.

His Honor : Would you have seen them if any had been present ?

Witness : I should have expected to find extensive disease of the kidneys, which even the decayed state of the body would have shown.

His Honor : Supposing you had known nothing of Captain Cain during life, and just examined the body, what would you have said apart from finding antimony ?

Witness : I should have said that he died from valvular disease of the heart.

His Honor : Is not this the case : that a man may have died of antimony poisoning and yet on *post mortem* examination you may not find a quantity enough to constitute a fatal dose ?

Witness : I might not find any poison.

His Honor : A man might be poisoned by antimony and yet you find no antimony in him ?

Witness : Many cases are recorded of persons who have died from poisoning and no poison found after death.

Mr Chapman : Of antimony ?

Witness : Of arsenic.

His Honor : Did you make any calculation of the quantity of antimony you found ?

Witness : I did not.

To Mr Haggitt : All the blood I found in the body and in the heart was in a fluid state. That is not the case where death results from gradual failure of the vital parts. If it had been a case of death from gradual failure of the vital parts I should have expected to find clots. Fluidity of the blood is given as one of the signs of antimonial poisoning. We found a considerable quantity of blood in the pleural cavity, and should find that in every case of slow death. That blood was accumulating during the last few hours of life.

Mr Haggitt : If sickness was caused by disease of the kidneys, what would be the particular cause of the sickness in such a case ?—It would be what is called uremic poisoning.

If uremic poisoning existed, would one expect to find a urinous odour in the breath which would be pretty well marked ?

Witness : I believe that is always the case in uremic poisoning, and it would be very noticeable. With sickness the result of uremic poisoning you would probably have constant nausea. A man who was suffering from uremic poisoning would not be likely to enjoy his breakfast. I think there was no uremic poisoning in Captain Cain's case. From what I have heard Captain Cain could eat food in the morning, he had turns of appetite and was not squeamish all day, and the sickness came on after meals. These symptoms were inconsistent with uremic poisoning. The dropsy I think was caused by heart disease. I should say the symptoms described during the last hours of Captain Cain's life—drowsiness, &c—were caused by the gradual failure of the system. At the *post mortem* the bronchial tubes appeared healthy, and I think the fluid in the pleura and the state of the heart accounted for the cough. The defective heart action would lead to the accumulation of fluid in the lower part of the lungs, and this fluid would get into the bronchial tubes. There was no enlargement or disease of the glands of the bowel or belly.

Cross-examined by Mr Chapman : The glands of the belly did not stand out as they would have done if diseased. I did not examine the kidneys microscopically. It was impossible to do so; they were too soft. I did not examine the brain. I did not open the head because we should have found the brain in a state of fluidity. I have examined bodies after interment both in Prague and in Aberdeen. The only case I could recall without my notes was one child. In that case the body had been buried a few weeks. There was another case in which the body of a man laid under the mud at the bottom of a mill pond for four months. It did not pass through my mind at the *post mortem* that there had been uremic poisoning. I looked at the kidney and could not discover advanced disease of the kidney. So far as I could judge the kidneys appeared healthy. There would be no change to any material extent in the size of the kidney in the state it was in after death. A medical-legal examination in a case like this is a blank sheet to me; I have to find out what is written on it. The kidneys were of about the normal size. We do not find the kidneys contracted in all cases of disease. In some cases of Bright's disease they are larger than the normal size; in some smaller, and in some cases they are of normal size. I went to the *post mortem* without any idea of the cause of death, but mainly to search for a particular irritant poison. The object of the *post mortem* was to remove certain parts so as to search for poison and also to discover the cause of death. The body was only partly removed from the coffin. I think I had information as to the symptoms during life before making the *post mortem* ; but I should not note them down. We did not make notes at the *post mortem*. It has been my practice to take notes at the *post mortem* table. I used generally to dictate my notes to some assistant. I noted the external appearances first, and then completed the whole of the internal examinations before taking notes, but made the notes before closing the body. I did not dictate notes to anyone on this occasion. I followed the English system of not taking the notes. I found that a written formal report is not necessary in English courts, and therefore did not take notes. My private opinion is that the Scotch system is the best. I suppose when a person comes to where loose customs are adopted he follows them.

Mr Chapman : Is that the kind of doctrine you propose to inculcate here ?—I find the custom prevalent in English legal forms, and I cannot alter it; at least I am not aware that I can.

You admit that the English practice is a loose one ?—Yes.

Are you aware of the actual practice of the best men in making *post mortems* in England and in New Zealand ?—I do not know anything about New Zealand. I know that it is not the practice in England to make notes at a *post mortem*.

Do you say you know it is not the practice of careful investigators to make notes as they proceed at a *post mortem*?—It is not the usual practice among English medical men.

But you say it is in Scotland?—Yes, and in Prague the notes are taken in duplicate. I have been in America. The law there is much the same as it is in England and the colonies.

Mr Chapman : Do you agree with this caution: "These examinations (*post mortem* examinations) should be made with more than usual care. The external inspection of the body and the examination of all the viscera should be thorough and detailed. Every appearance should be noted at the time, and nothing left to the memory"?—So far I agree with him, if the body is fresh, and if there is any object for examining minutely; but every medical jurist is accustomed to take his own way. I have never failed to remember for month's afterwards any case I have seen. I can trust my memory as to details, and it is not necessary for me to take notes.

You think that confidence supersedes a direction of this kind?—I do.

In Scotland you were of a different opinion?—I followed the practice there. Considering I had been working from half-past 7 until half-past 1 the following morning, I think I was quite excusable for leaving my notes that night, and besides there were no conveniences for taking notes there. I have looked over them to make sure they were all there. I never found yet that my memory failed me in a case of this sort. I made notes three or four days ago and gave them to the Crown prosecutor. I have not seen them since. Dr Hogg looked over them and he concurred. The phrase "The notes which I have used I made only a few days ago" must mean the notes which have been used by Mr Haggitt, were made two or three days ago. Dr Hogg looked over the notes, and there were one or two points which he thought had not been described perhaps fully enough, and we made one or two trifling additions. My examination yesterday was made wider than my notes. The examination this morning proceded on the notes Dr Hogg and I had signed. I was examined this morning on a supplemental note. Had you asked for the same notes I would have given them.

Mr Chapman : Would you in the middle of your examination be prepared to give notes to the defence in order that you might be examined upon them?—I see no reason why I should not. An expert is not here to give evidence for a particular side, but to bring out the facts of the case.

Were these notes asked for or were they given voluntarily?—They were asked for.

Witness continued: For my description of these *post mortem* appearances, I rely on my memory for four months. In natural death from failure of the heart I should expect to find clots in every case of slow death. I did not form an absolute opinion from that that death was unnatural, but there was something unusual about it; it was suspicious. Uremic poisoning ends in coma. The smell of urine from the breath would probably be noticed by the patient and complained of. I have seen a case in which antimony has been used with benefit for asthma,

but never heard of it being used with cigarettes. The druggist knows nothing about disease, and is incompetent to advise. Both doctors and druggist sometimes make experiments. A cigarette containing antimony might poison by contact with the lips. We did not search for vegetable poisons. They were mentioned to us, but I said decay was so far advanced, the body had been so long there, that I put it to him, "Is it any use looking for them?" That was after forming my own opinion that it was useless to look for vegetable poisons.

Mr Chapman : That is the position you take—one of extreme modesty?—No; one of courtesy.

You did not intend to follow Dr Hogg's opinion?—If Dr Hogg had said we must look for it we would have looked for it.

Witness continued : I do not say with regard to all alkaloids that I would not search for them. My opinion is that it would be of no use looking for them after death, but we did not finally abandon the idea of searching for these poisons until we found antimony. If we had not found antimony we should have sought for other poisons. It was our duty to find a deadly poison, and also to seek for the cause of death. I should not expect to find colchicum or atropia a long time after death. It would surprise me to find that experts had found those poisons a considerable period after death. If you get a perfectly fresh body you might find those poisons.

To Mr Haggitt : The notes were prepared at your request, and for your use. I was not examined in this case till yesterday. In Scotland, the practice is to make a report of the *post mortem*, which report must be made within three days. Except in Scotland, that practice does not prevail. The decision not to search for vegetable poisons was made during the *post mortem*, and during the analysis. On the last occasion Dr Black was present, and was consulted.

Dr Black deposed : I am a professor of chemistry at the University of Otago, a doctor of science of the University of Edinburgh, and extra-mural lecturer in chemistry for the Universities of Edinburgh, Glasgow, and Aberdeen. I recollect Constable Daly bringing me a box to Dunedin on August 18 last. It was a wooden box, closed and sealed. The box contained several articles, all of which I analysed. I was careful to see that everything I used for the purpose was clean and free from antimony. The first thing that I analysed was the contents of a small phial, which I found to contain a soluble salt of antimony—tartar emetic, or tartarised antimony. The next thing I analysed were two pockets cut from trousers. I analysed the two together, and found antimony in some soluble form—certainly tartar emetic. Next I examined a packet of tartar emetic from Gunn's, said to have been found in trousers pocket. I found it was tartar emetic. I also found a small packet of powder, found on the floor of the dining room. It contained tartar emetic. A bottle said to be found in Hall's bedroom contained a solution of tartar emetic. A small bottle containing a white powder I found to be common saltpetre, otherwise known as nitrate of potash. Next I examined a small bottle containing weak lime water, and a small packet which contained bismuth powders. The next thing I examined was a bottle containing brandy for injections. I examined it, but found no antimony. The next exhibit was labelled " Ice water for sick room, prepared only for use there." It contained no antimony. A piece of cork which was cut lengthways I next examined. Some white powder was attached to it, which I found to be tartar emetic. Ice water taken from the cup, sealed by Dr Macintyre, was then analysed. It was a solution of tartar emetic, at the rate of eight grains to the ounce. Vomit, labelled 12th August, was found to contain antimony. A bottle said to contain urine passed on the 12th August was also found to contain antimony. From Constable Egan I received a packet containing five articles. There was first some vomit of August 13, which was found to contan antimony. There were four other articles—a colander, three pieces of flannel, a piece of gauze cloth, and a piece of sacking—which did not contain antimony. From Dr Macintyre in his own laboratory at Timaru I received various bottles. This was on September 4. In fæces of August 17 I found antimony; in fæces of August 19 I found antimony, also of August 12. In urine of August 18 I found antimony. With Dr Ogston I analysed urine of August 19 and August 24, in which we found antimony. All these analyses were conducted in the university laboratory at Dunedin. From Constable Daly I received another box on September 16 at the laboratory, Dunedin. It contained a bottle containing brandy, said to be for injection. Dr Ogston and I examined it. We found no antimony, but found colchicin. We also received a bottle of urine of August 20, and found antimony. In another bottle, containing fæces of August 12, we found antimony. There were two other bottles labelled " Urine of September 13 and 14." We examined for antimony for scientific purposes. There was a bare suspicion of antimony, but nothing to swear to. A bottle labelled " August 15," containing urine, was found to contain antimony. There was also a bottle of vomit containing antimony. I analysed some cigarettes which we got from Inspector Broham in Christchurch. We tested them for antimony, but did not get any. Of the first 15 Dr Hogg repeated the analysis in four cases, and the results corresponded with the results I obtained. We tried several tests in each case. The exhibits were always locked up, and I kept the key myself. Dr Ogston and Dr Hogg brought four bottles for analysis on the evening of the 28th of September last. Those were the four bottles I saw in court yesterday. I offered to put the laboratory at Dr Ogston's disposal, but he insisted upon my making the analysis. I consented, and considered myself responsible for the analysis. Dr Hogg assisted me greatly—was always with me; and Dr Ogston also assisted. Drs Ogston and Hogg made independent analyses, and I saw the result of their analyses. The bottles were clear glass and wide-mouthed, closed with a cork and sealed with Dr Ogston's seal. Dr Ogston also handed to me for analysis

a quantity of earth, which was tested for antimony, but I did not find any in it. The bottles were labelled in Roman capitals—I, II, III, IV. No. I contained the bladder, kidneys, urine, and portion of small intestines ; No. II contained a dark fluid from the lateral cavity of the chest ; No. III, the stomach and part of the small intestines ; No IV contained part of the larger intestines, the rectum, liver, and spleen. There was fluid in each bottle. No. I bottle was tested as follows : On September 28 a portion of the liquid was acidified with hydrochloric acid and boiled for 10 minutes with a slip of clean copper, and at the end of 15 minutes it was examined and found coated with a violet-coloured deposit. The same liquid was boiled with another slip of copper for 10 minutes with the same result. Another slip of copper was added, and the material boiled again for 10 minutes, producing a very slight tinge of violet on the copper. When the second and third slips of copper were added, the first remained in the fluid, and when the third was added they all remained in. The violet tint corresponded with that which a small quantity of antimony gives by the same treatment. We examined the three slips by the permanganate test, but making a mistake in the process the result was of no value. The mistake was in not filtering before adding hydrochloric acid. The mistake was mine. The same tests were applied to liquids from the same bottle on the following day, the 29th, several slips of copper being used, and the permanganate test being properly applied, the slips were coloured violet, and the sulphuretted hydrogen gave a small orange precipitate. Liquid from No. II was boiled for 10 minutes with hydrochloric acid, and slips of clean copper put in, and when examined at the end of 15 minutes a very slight dimness of the copper was observed. The copper was replaced in the same liquid and boiled again for 10 minutes. At the end of half an hour from the commencement of this boiling the copper was examined, and found to have a slight but decided violet tint. Liquid from No. III bottle, together with scrapings from the coating of the stomach, treated in the same way, gave a slight but decided violet tint. The tin test was applied to the liquid from each of the four bottles in the following way :—A small piece of tinfoil was dropped in a part of the liquor in a clean porcelain cup, and the tinfoil was very slightly dimmed in the course of half-an-hour, and had become of a dark leaden hue at the end of 12 hours—it was quite black—pointing to a trace of antimony or something else, establishing the absence of a large quantity of antimony in the article tested. On October 3 I collected the orange precipitates before referred to, dissolved them in strong hot hydrochloric acid, and applied the galvanic test, and found antimony. Reinsch's test was repeated on the following day, September 29, and the results confirmed the first analysis. We also tested part of the contents of the bottles by the Fresenius and Von Babo process as follows :— Dr Hogg cut up in the finest shreds parts of the solids in No. I bottle into a clean porcelain dish ; digested the same with liquid from No. I bottle in a porcelain basin, with strong hydrochloric acid and successive portions of powdered chlorate potash We burned over a Bunsen burner till the chlorate was decomposed, the solid parts dissolved into a yellowish liquid, and the free chlorien expelled. We then let the liquor cool, filtered through a wet filter, and removed most of the fatty matter by agitation with ether, separating the ethermal solution by an ordinary glass separator. We then warmed the separated solution till all traces of ether were expelled and again filtered it. Then treated with sulphuretted hydrogen sample, and very soon got a yellow colour, and afterwards a cloudy orange precipitate. Compared this precipitate with some similar precipitate got by sulphur-etted hydrogen, with solutions of antimony, at various stages of dilution. We repeated the hydrochloric test on a second portion of the same solution with a like result. We treated parts of Nos. II and IV bottles together—namely, part of black liquid of No. II, and part of the liver and spleen of No. IV bottle, cut up by Dr Hogg, and digested as before with hydrochloric acid, till the solids were destroyed; but on applying Reinsch's test to part of the solution, we found free chloriue. After repeated efforts to clear the solution from chlorine, we changed our mode of procedure. We boiled the remainder of the solution down to dryness, and charred the residue in a close platinum vessel. We then drenched the mass in strong hydrochloric acid, heating it over a Bunsen burner. We then diluted it with water and filtered it, and applied the following test:—We dropped a small piece of tinfoil into it, and this was blackened in half-an-hour. We then applied Reinsch's test, and the copper had a violet tint in 15 minutes. To a third portion we applied the galvanic test, and got a very slight darkening of the platinum wire in 12 hours, indicating minute traces of antimony or something else. We then took parts of Nos. 1, and 4 bottles, and applied Von Babo's test, viz., from No. 1 bottle part of the small intestines; from No. 3 bottle part of the stomach and duodenum, and from No. 4 bottle part of the cæcum and rectum. Dr Hogg cut up the solids, and these were digested with liquid from the same bottles with strong hydrochloric acid and chlorate of potash. After destroying the solids, decomposing the chlorate, and boiling off the free chlorine, we removed the fatty matters by agitatum with ether. We tested the residuary solution in the following way:—To about four-fifths of it we added sulphuretted hydrogen, passing a strong current of gas through it, and got first a yellow colour, then an orange precipitate. We applied the tin test. The tin was slightly darkened in about 20 minutes, but not quite black in half-an-hour, and quite black, with a slight deposit around it in 12 hours. We boiled another portion with a piece of clean copper, and got a slight violet tint iu 15 minutes. On the Friday following (October 1) I applied a quantitative test to the contents of the four bottles, to find approximately but very roughly the quantity of antimony. With this view I collected the two orange precipitates referred to above, and entered by me in the depositions in pages 79 and 81. Washed them, dried them, and weighed them. Found the weight to be ·009 grains, equal to ·1388 of a grain of sulphide antimony, which represents about ·271 of a grain of tartar emetic. I assumed this to have been got from one-eighth of the contents of the whole four bottles. Now that multiplied by eight would give a shade over two grains of tartar emetic for the whole of the stuff analysed. On the same day, September 29, after weighing the sulphide of antimony, I further identified it by resolving strong hydrochloric acid, and getting the white oxychloride of antimony. By the addition of water this white oxychloride was found to be soluble in a strong solution of tartaric acid. From this solution I reprecipitated an orange precipitate by the addition of sulphurated hydrogen. On October 3 I identified the black powder referred to above as accompanying the tin by washing it and dissolving it in strong hot hydrochloric acid, and then reprecipitating as au orange precipitate by sulphuretted hydrogen. There were also some tests by the process of dialysis. The dialysis performed by Drs Hogg, Ogston, and myself on September 30 was as follows:—We boiled part of the contents of bottles Nos. II and IV with strong hydrochloric acid, and after cooling and diluting with water, we placed the liquid in a dialyser. At the end of from 10 to 15 hours we examined the dialysate by Reinsch's test, and got a slight violet tint on the copper at the end of 10 minutes. We applied the same test to the residuum still left in the dialyser, and got a decided violet tint. To these two slips of copper was tried the permanganate test, and got with sulphurated hydrogen a yellow solution, deepening in standing to an orange precipitate. We also dialysed a portion of the liquid contents of bottles 1 and 2 without previously adding hydrochloric acid, and got similar results. We then dialysed at the same time portions both of solids and liquids from bottles Nos. 1, 2, 3, and 4, after boiling with strong hydrochloric acid, and got similar results. We applied heat to one of the violet-tinted copper slips referred to above, and at a black heat there was no change. At a red heat the violet deposit disappeared in a small puff of white fume, which is characteristic of antimony. Arsenic would have gone off at a lower temperature. Know of nothing else that would do the same except antimony. This was a confirmatory test to make ourselves quite sure. We tested the earth bottles for nothing but antimony. We resolved that it would be useless to look for any organic poison, owing to the length of time which had elapsed since the death of Captain Cain. We did not analyse any of the solids separately—that is to say, any individual solids. The tests showed only very small, but decided, quantities of antimony.

To Mr Chapman : The proportion of antimony in tartar emetic is about 36 per cent. This process of dialysing must, I should say, be very similar to the action of the human body—very

48

like liquids passed through membrane into the bladder.

Mr Chapman: Suppose pieces of the body were brought together in one bottle with these liquids, or that they were put together and liquid added to them, what would happen?

Witness: You would have a transfusion of the liquids and it would represent a mixture of the whole.

For instance, if portions containing the urine and urinary bladder and part of the intestines were put together you would not expect to be able to get the liquid again and call it urine?

No; it would be mixed up.

No further questions were asked Dr Black in cross-examination.

Mr Haggitt: That is the last witness, your Honor, that we propose to call.

Mr Chapman objected to several of the exhibits connected with the previous case in which Hall was concerned being put in.

His Honor (to Mr Haggitt): Do you think they are necessary to your case?

Mr Haggitt: I do not know that they are. I will leave it to your Honor. You know what the cases are.

His Honor: I must say that if the other evidence about Mrs Hall is admissible, it seems to me logically to follow that these exhibits are admissible also. But as I said before, the question of the admissibility of the whole has never yet been decided by a court for Crown cases reserved, and there has been, as you know, one case in which the whole of such evidence was held not admissible. There is also this to be borne in mind: that in one of the most celebrated poisoning trials that ever took place—that of Palmer,—in which the most eminent criminal judge of the day and the most eminent criminal advocate were engaged, evidence of the kind suggested was not brought forward or attempted to be, although in Palmer's case true bills had been found, and although from the facts of the case—strychnine not having been found in the body—any evidence of the circumstances of these two deaths that could have been got in would have been important. The question was not discussed, but the fact that the evidence was not brought in under those circumstances makes it worthy of some consideration. I think on the whole, from every point of view, the ends of justice will be best served for reasons, which I may give hereafter, that the question of the admissibility of the whole of this evidence should be reserved. That course does not affect your conduct of the case, Mr Haggitt?

Mr Haggitt: I shall be guided by your Honor.

His Honor: If you think it essential——

Mr Haggitt: It is clearly not absolutely essential.

His Honor: No. I will admit the exhibits and reserve the point. I admit I have some hesitation about it. You are quite right, of course, to tender them, because in the case of the Queen v. Eason they were held admissible. So far as the evidence that has already been admitted is concerned there can be no question. Although the point has been reserved, it was

proper, from the authorities, that the evidence should be tendered and received at the trial.

Mr Haggitt: If you think I should not, I will not press the matter.

His Honor: I do not say that it would be indiscreet. Of course if you do not tender them nothing can be said about them in your address.

Mr Haggitt: That is so. It is perfectly manifest the use that I could make of them.

His Honor: Quite so.

Mr Haggitt: If you think I should not risk putting them in I shall not.

His Honor: It seems to me that it is carrying the question in the cases of the Queen v. Flanagan and the Queen v. Gearin a step farther than they go.

Mr Haggitt: Mr Justice Butt merely said he should hesitate to admit such evidence as evidence of motive. If your Honor thinks there is any doubt about it I will not press it, but leave them out. They are not essential.

His Honor: If not, I think it would be prudent not to press them.

Mr Haggitt: That is the case, then, your Honor.

Mr Chapman: Does the Crown not call Buchanan?

Mr Haggitt: As far as I can understand, he was not there at the time of the death. He took one or two nights' nursing only. We have made inquiries, and the result is that he can say absolutely nothing of the slightest value to the case.

Mr Chapman: Of the slightest value to the Crown.

Mr Haggitt: To the case, I said.

His Honor: His name is not mentioned in the indictment. I do not see that the Crown is under a necessity to call him. Do you call evidence, Mr Chapman?

Mr Chapman: Yes, your Honor.

THE DEFENCE.

Mr Denniston said: May it please your Honor. Gentlemen of the jury,—The evidence for the prosecution being closed, it now becomes my duty to lay before you briefly the evidence proposed to be called to strengthen the position in which the evidence led for the Crown has left us. That position is, I think, that the Crown has absolutely and entirely failed to establish the issue which it was its duty to prove. It is no part of my duty now to attempt to go into any details as to the evidence in this case, or to anticipate the defence which will be afterwards made on behalf of the accused. It will be the duty of my learned friend Mr Chapman, who leads in this case, at, I hope, a no distant date to go fully into the details and sum up the case for the defence, and I am content to leave that duty in his hands. All I shall do is to open briefly the general nature of the defence. The prosecution undertakes to establish three things—first, that antimony was found in the body of Captain Cain; secondly, that the administration of antimony necessarily accelerated his death; and thirdly, that such antimony is conclusively and incontestably shown to have been given to him by Thomas Hall, the prisoner. As to the first point, that antimony was found in the body, we can necessarily offer no evidence. The whole manipulation of the body and the details of the examination have been in the hands of the Crown, and we are virtually in their hands as far as that part of the case is concerned. On the second proposition, that his death was accelerated by antimony, presuming it to have been administered, we do intend to call medical evidence. That point, although it may be to some extent abstract and technical, is vital to the prosecution. It is not so to us, of course, because you may come to an affirmative conclusion upon it and yet leave 'untouched the main ground on which we rely. Although it is an abstract and technical point, and not one which a jury generally favours being relied on, still there are circumstances which we cannot affect to ignore, which I think will induce you to attach some weight to that point, and at any rate to approach it with an unprejudiced and unbiassed mind. The evidence for the prosecution shows conclusively that the death was originally attributed to natural causes by all who noticed it. It is now attempted, long after the event, when the memories of men have altered and circumstances have been forgotten, to establish a different conclusion. It is desired, on the strength of a careless diagnosis and a slovenly *post mortem* examination, entirely based on a foregone conclusion as to the real cause of death, to establish that this death was necessarily and conclusively accelerated by the fact of antimony having been administered. We do not pretend on our part to produce witnesses to speak with that certainty and confidence which was characteristic of some of the witnesses for the Crown. We shall say that the evidence of those witnesses outside mere expert evidence has been clearly in our favour as to the necessary certainty of such inferences. And our evidence will be directed to this effect: That considering the physical condition of Captain Cain, the absolute uncertainty as to the time, the quantity, and the circumstances of the administration of antimony, and the conditions of death, it is impossible to prove conclusively that death was accelerated by these means. In this case we are not asked to, and cannot prove a negative. It is not for us to prove that death was not accelerated, and that without the administration of antimony the deceased must have died on a particular date; it is for the other side to establish absolutely that death was, and must have been, so accelerated—that he must have been alive after the date he was, but for the administration of antimony during his life. That is the proposition which we say the other side have entirely failed to establish, and the proposition as to which we shall bring medical evidence. As to what that evidence is, I need not trouble you with details; it is sufficient to say that the witnesses will be taken over the ground that was gone over with such confidence by the witnesses for the Crown. They will describe how slovenly and careless some of the processes were, and

say that the results stated cannot be arrived at. We say that it is unnecessary and impossible for us to establish that this antimony if administered was not a depressent. It is not for us to prove that the administration could be judicious, or could have a good effect. It is simply enough for us to show that there are no data—or data so imperfect as to make it impossible for any person to prove that death must have been accelerated by antimony. As regards the third point, as to the alleged administration by Hall, we are also necessarily circumscribed, and for this reason : The Crown have not pretended to suggest any proved instance of administration. They rely on a mass of indirect circumstances, pointing, I say, not even to the inference of any administration by Hall more than by any other person. They simply content themselves with showing in wearisome detail the whole circumstances of the last few months before Cain's death, and ask you to infer that someone must have poisoned him and that the poisoner must have been Thomas Hall. I venture to say that neither I nor you know how, where, in what vehicle, or in what manner Hall can possibly be said to have administered poison. The first suggestion was that it was in whisky, then champagne, then cough mixture, and I suppose the next will be jellies. There is no possibility of saying from the case in what, or at what time, Hall is supposed to have administered poison. Every point raised we have met, and we have in fact proved that every symptom on which the other side relied as being evidence of poisoning existed at times and places and under circumstances inconsistent with the administration of poison by Hall. But what the Crown practically relies on is placing before you a mass of details as to the life of Captain Cain, showing that Hall might have been there and could have and might have administered poison; and on the strength of that, and trusting to the prejudice and ill will excited by circumstances which we cannot affect to ignore, inducing you to find a verdict which certainly no evidence before you could possibly lead you to give. Because on the evidence already given as to the circumstances of Cain's death, the manner his meals were given, his symptoms, and the manner of his attendance and nursing, it is impossible for you, apart from the shadow sought to be thrown over the case by other incidents and events, to come to the conclusion that there is even a suggestion that Hall more than any other person had anything to do with the administration of poison. The question of motive will also be dealt with by my learned friend. It is enough for me to show that there has been an absolute breakdown in the case opened by the Crown prosecutor. Where the Crown alleges that Cain did not consent we have proved that he did; where it was alleged that we should benefit we have shown that not only did we not benefit but we ourselves conferred the benefit; and practically you will see that the callous destruction of this old man imputed to us would have been absolutely resultless, and must have been known to us to be so at the time. We shall now confine ourselves to calling some evidence to add to the circumstances in our favour brought out by the Crown's evidence as to the details of the death, sickness, &c. There is one point in this branch of the case, as to whether Hall was himself the administrator of the poison, that I want to refer to. Incidentally the evidence alleges the purchase of a book on poisons at a given date and under given circumstances. Now it is not disputed that Hall had a book of the sort and had studied the subject. It has been proved that he had the necessity to; for one reason because he was in the habit of administering narcotics to himself, and for another because he was in the habit of dealing with certain disorders with poisonous elements, and it is a proved fact that he asserted that he used antimony for this purpose. But is it not an immense leap from this to prove that he was at the time studying the subject for the purpose of planning a murder of this extraordinary nature? The evidence relied on as regards this book ("Taylor on Poisons") is not so much that he purchased it, as that he wrote in it a wrong date with a sinister design. The whole strength of that point, depends upon the identification by the witness Hutton of the particular volume put in evidence. The question is not whether or not on that date Hall purchased from Hutton a volume relating to poisons. The point is his purchasing this individual volume and making this particular alteration in the date of purchase. This point turns upon the question of how far you believe Hutton's identification of the book. Identification of one volume among a large edition issued by the same publisher can only be by some peculiar mark. Hutton saw the cogency of this, and pretended to swear to this very volume as the one he sold Hall—not from any writing, or mark or private note, but simply from its general resemblance to the book he sold; and when pressed he swore that he knew it by the particular abrasion you see here. You will see that in fact the whole book is greatly abraded and has seen strong service; and if Hutton is to be believed, it must have seen that service before it left him, because he has sworn that it presents very much the same appearance. Can you believe that is possible? He admits that he had not this particular identification in his mind when he sold the book: yet he pretends to recognise it by that abrasion, and for the first time, for no mention of it was made elsewhere. He also swore that its general condition was the same when sold. I ask you if during any number of years, simply remaining on the shelves of a bookseller, it could possibly have got into the condition in which this book is. I ask if such a conclusion is intelligent and possible. But Hutton was not content with that. He told you he identified it by the remains of a private mark, and by the remains of the price mark (18s 6d). I defy anyone with any microscope to detect one single detail of such marks as confirming him. I am content to leave it to you whether any trace of such marks can be discovered. I say, therefore, that on this alone, gentlemen, it would be impossible for you to believe him or to credit his evidence on the point. I may say, too, that we propose to call evidence to help you to believe

us. The men we shall produce cannot pretend to speak as to absolute identity—only such men as Mr Hutton can do that. But we shall call unimpeachable evidence that as far back as 1884—considerably before the date mentioned—a book of this size, "Taylor on Poisons" was in Hall's possession. We shall prove that it was in his possession in April, the month directly antecedent to his alleged purchase from Hutton. We shall prove that a book exactly similar was in his hands certainly two months before the date he is alleged to have purchased it. There is also one witness who will say—although not with absolute confidence—that his name was written in the book; but that is a detail. These facts will not prove absolutely that it was the same book; but you will be asked to say, first, is it likely that a man in possession of the book would first borrow and then buy another copy merely to excite suspicion? I omitted one inherent absurdity of Hutton's story. Is it likely Hall would purchase the book, and that the idea should pass through his mind: "I mean to use it to poison somebody; I may be arrested, and I shall now provide for that by putting a wrong date in the book, and I will do that in the face of the man I purchased it from, who can, if necessary, be called to prove it against me?" It would, I hope, require more evidence than that of Mr Hutton to prove this. This reasoning, if you believe it, will remove a point which, though comparatively unimportant, is of a nature to impress a jury somewhat unfavourably. Moreover it is an illustration of the manner in which details are piled up against an accused person, and how easily they are disposed of even after this lapse of time. We happen to be able to dispose of it in this instance, but we may not be in others. It also shows how easy it is, directly there is ill-feeling against a person, to turn, twist, and alter trifling circumstances to his disadvantage. This, you must bear in mind, has not been an honest inquiry into the circumstances of Cain's death. From the beginning the whole strength of the prosecution has been directed against this man alone. The Crown have directed their attention to one point, and ignored, as only police officials can ignore, everything tending in favour of the accused. What the result would have been had the inquiry been conducted differently I cannot say; but against this man only have all the resources of the Crown been directed, to give every incident the most sinister appearance and throw the whole mass of details before you, trusting that the ill-feeling and prejudice excited against the prisoner may lead you to colour every trifling incident until they may possibly produce belief in your minds. I cannot believe that even with this colour they can have this effect; but it is not my business to discuss that. My object has simply been to open to you—I hope at not too great length—the evidence it is proposed to call for the defence. Not that we rely upon it. We are strong enough in the weakness of the Crown. We call it to strengthen the conviction that the Crown's evidence must have created—viz., that they have fallen far short of that absolute certainty which alone could justify a verdict at your hands.

Mr Denniston then called Edward Wakefield, M.H.R., journalist, residing at Wellington, who said: I came down about this case. I know the accused Hall, and have known him intimately for a long time.

Mr Denniston: Do you remember on any occasion having seen a book on poisons in his hands?

Witness: In his hands?

Mr Denniston: Or in his house.

Witness: I remember seeing a book on poisons in his lodgings at Timaru during some part of 1884. It was "Taylor on Poisons." To the best of my recollection, it was on the chest of drawers in his bedroom.

Mr Denniston: Can you tell us any later date that you saw it?

Witness: I saw the same work some months later at his house. I think it must have been in April 1885. I had been to Australia for a visit and returned at the end of March, and arrived at Timaru in the first week of April. I know it was within a few days of my arrival, because I left again for Wellington at the end of April. I went out to Hall's house at Kingsdown, and I noticed the book with others on the shelf. I was alone and I remember taking it down from the shelf and reading it. When Hall came into the room I spoke to him about a large mastiff of mine which had the mange, and said something about having it poisoned. I referred to a passage in the book about prussic acid being applied externally to the nervous membrane. I asked Hall if it was not a law book, and he said he had picked it up in Dunedin a year or two before. That was in April 1885. The book produced is the same work, and it was very like this volume. I have no doubt about the book being "Taylor on Poisons."

To Mr Haggitt: I could not say that this book produced is the identical volume, but it is the same work. I do not recollect looking inside the covers, or seeing any writing. I looked at the index, not I think at the beginning or end of the book. I know Hall had a similar volume in 1884, and it was when he was laid up with sciatica, because I went to see him.

Benjamin Daniel Hibbard deposed: I know the accused Thomas Hall. At one time he lodged with me, and left me in 1885. While he was with me I knew of his possession of "Taylor on Poisons." That was in 1884, or it might be 1883. I went to see him one night in his room and saw the book lying on the bed. I took the book up and looked at it. I have an impression that his name was written in it obliquely, at the back part of it. I have an impression that "T. Hall, Dunedin" was in it.

To Mr Haggitt: I may never have seen the book produced before; but I did see a book "Taylor on Poisons" in Hall's possession in the winter of 1883 or 1884.

To Mr Denniston: Before the trial in Christchurch I informed the police I had seen the book. It was known I had seen the book, and

I was subpœnaed, but was not called. The police saw me about it, and it was the only subject on which I could give evidence.

To Mr Haggitt: I saw Inspector Broham and Detective Kirby, but I do not know whether it was before or after the trial. I told the police I could not identify the book. I saw the counsel for the defence. The day the first case was on in court in Timaru, I had a communication from Mrs Hall, asking if I knew of such a book. I saw her and told her I knew of it, and everybody knew of it after that, I suppose. I never kept this fact secret from the prisoner's counsel.

George Buchanan (a settler residing at Timaru), deposed: I knew the late Captain Cain intimately, I sat up with him near the time of his death. I commenced to sit up with him on the 21st of January, and sat up with him alternate nights to the day of his death. I was a large part of the time alone with Cain, but could get the nurses if wanted. In the early part of the night Captain Cain was chatty. His breathing was short and sterturous. I noticed swelling about his face and under the eyes. I did not notice any delirium. He did not sleep for more than 20 minutes or half an hour at a time. The cough generally waked him up, and he used to ask for his cough mixture. The captain used sometimes to shake his head after taking the mixture as if he did not like it. He was not sick after the cough mixture. During the night he used to have jellies and biscuit. He took whisky and it did not disagree with him. He also had champagne taken from a bottle by a syphon. I gave him whisky from the stand on the table. I took some whisky myself from the stand, and it never had any effect upon me at any time. I was summoned by the police at the preliminary inquiry, and told the police I had sat up and had never seen Cain sick. I mentioned to the police that I had given Cain whisky and had never seen him sick. I told Mr White the evidence I could give, and he said they would not want to call me. Cain was cheerful and would talk about old times when he woke up. That was so on the night of the 27th.

To Mr Haggitt: I used to go between 8 and 9 o'clock. Very often Wren and Kay, the nurses, would be there. When they were in the room together, it was for the purpose of raising Captain Cain from his bed and attending to him. Sometimes one of them would sleep in the room on the sofa, and one was always within call. I was there the whole of four nights and never saw Cain sick, and if he had been sick I should have noticed his sickness. Each night I gave him something to eat and something to drink, and he was not sick. The whisky and water agreed with him. I think he had it every night twice or three times. Cain also had his cough mixture, and he seemed not to like it. The cough mixture did not make Cain sick. I remember giving Cain champagne on more than one occasion. I drew the champagne into an ordinary tumbler. I have seen Captain Cain have broth or soup brought from the kitchen. I did not see very much difference on the 27th, the last time I was there. I usually left about daybreak. Towards the latter part of the night, from 2 or 3 o'clock to 5, he used to sleep. That was his longest sleep. I cannot say what nights Kay was there, but he was there I think mostly every night.

Mr Haggitt : If Kay has told us there was no night that he was not sick three or four times, or perhaps more?—I should say he had made a mistake decidedly, unless he called it sickness when Captain Cain after coughing spat out phlegm into a pocket handkerchief.

Witness continued : I heard of Captain Cain being sick before he took to his bedroom. I heard of that frequently. Captain Cain to the last was cheerful as a sick man would be.

Mr Haggitt : Have you told the police you could not give any evidence at all?—I asked the police when they summoned me what they were bringing me down for, and said that my evidence would not go for much, I should say.

Was it not the fact that you did not want to give evidence?—It is the fact that most people don't want to give evidence.

Witness continued : I may have said that I did not want to give evidence. I occupied a cottage belonging to the prisoner's father. I have been in Timaru lately, but not in that cottage. Since the case came on I have been principally up country.

To Mr Denniston : I have never been very intimate with the prisoner. After his child was born I called at his house and was asked to stay to dinner. That was the first time I exchanged twenty words with Hall. Captain Cain was an old friend of mine. I have known him since I landed in Timaru. It was at his request I went to sit up with him.

Ethel Morris deposed : I was one of the bridesmaids at Mr Hall's marriage. I was in Timaru a little before that and lived at Woodlands from 12th May to 11th July. During that time I saw Captain Cain vomiting twice. I heard of him being sick at other times, and saw a basin beside his chair on three occasions.

This witness was not cross-examined.

Mr Chapman stated that any of the other witnesses he had to call would be under examination about two hours.

His Honor said he was sorry for it, but the jury would have to be kept together until Monday.

Mr Haggitt suggested that there was no reason why the jury should not be taken a drive on Sunday.

The Foreman thought they might occupy the top of a tramcar for a part of the day, and so get the benefit of fresh air. That would be preferable to staying in an hotel all day.

Mr Chapman said that in Christchurch the jury had a drag supplied to them on the order of the judge, and were driven to Sumner. It would, he thought, be better to place a drag at their disposal than to allow them to go in a public vehicle.

His Honor said it was very desirable that the health and strength of the jury should be seen to, and if a drag had been provided for them before he saw no reason why it should not be done again. The sheriff would be directed to make suitable arrangements for taking the jury out.

The court adjourned shortly after 5 p.m.

MONDAY, JANUARY 31.

SEVENTH DAY OF THE TRIAL.

Joseph Edwards (manager at Hallenstein Brothers, Invercargill) deposed : I was working at Timaru for Mr Slater, and knew Captain Cain about June, July, or August 1885. Captain Cain during some time in those months came into the shop to make some purchases and became sick, vomiting very much.

Cross-examined : At the end of October I left for Christchurch for two months, and previously to that I was travelling into the country a good deal. The sickness occurred after Hall's marriage, and was not later than September.

Edward William Alexander, physician and surgeon, deposed : I have been practising in Dunedin for a good many years, and had practised for six or eight years previously. I heard the evidence given by Dr Macintyre in this case describing the symptoms of Captain Cain's illness. I also heard the description of the symptoms on the last day Dr Macintyre saw him. I heard the evidence of Stubbs and Kay. With those data before me I can say that so far as described Captain Cain's death was not inconsistent with a natural cause. The evidence was not altogether inconsistent with death by uremic poisoning. I could not draw any certain inference as to whether Captain Cain was probably or possibly suffering from Bright's disease. Uremic poisoning might occur in any form of Bright's disease or through any congestion of the kidneys where excretion is difficult Bright's disease is a degenerative condition of the kidneys, in which the albuminous element of the blood is poured out with the urine. Uremia is exceptional; it does not occur in all kidney diseases, but is an occasional natural result. Although it is but occasional, it is frequent enough to be quite familiar to physicians of experience. Some of the symptoms described point in the direction of uremic poisoning. When death results from that cause, the uremic poisoning usually produces stupor, sickness, and slight convulsive movements. The chronic form is often intermittent and usually terminates fatally. The odour in the breath is not necessarily discoverable in uremic poisoning. In cases of kidney disease death comes about from exhaustion, or from inflammation of some other part, hemorrhage of the stomach or of the brain. Hemorrhage of the brain would cause appoplexy ; slowly or rapidly, the patient would become insensible, and there would be stertorious breathing. When hemorrhage has occurred in the brain it is readily discernible by post mortem examination. The mode of Cain's death was not absolutely inconsistent with apoplexy of the kind I have mentioned, but the indications were not sufficiently marked to enable me to speak with absolute certainty. The data were insufficient to enable me to give a decided opinion. There was nothing in the symptoms attending Cain's death as described by Dr Macintyre, and Stubbs and Kay, distinctively suggestive of antimonial poisoning. The vomiting and purging spoken of as occurring previously were consistent with antimonial poisoning, but some of the symptoms of antimonial poisoning were absent. A single large dose of antimony produces persistent vomiting with great depression, &c., usually death. When vomiting is produced by antimony it is severe, and accompanied by retching. Antimony is still used in medicine, but very little in general practice. It is one of the best remedies in subduing brain excitement in mania. It also acts as a sedative by repressing excitement of the nervous system. In seeking the cause of death in a case of the kind I might have made a *post mortem* examination. I heard the evidence of the *post mortem*, and understood Dr Ogston to say that the main object was to seek for metallic poison. I have made a good many *post mortems*, but not as an expert. I think an examination of the brain would have shown whether there had been hemorrhage in the brain or not. I observed that no microscopic examination of the tissues of the kidney was made, and I cannot say whether it could have been made, and can hardly say what I would have done; but I think I should have opened the brain. I think I should have limited myself to a rough examination of the whole of the body. I might have handed the kidneys to someone who had special microscopic knowledge for examination. I do not attach much importance to absence of clot from the heart, as that occurs in |so many cases, and I should attach no importance to it as a symptom of poisoning. It would not be a circumstance tending to negative the inference that the death was a natural one. I agree with the opinion read from Orth's work on pathology, that "coagulation may be incomplete or entirely wanting in consequence either of diminution in the amount of fibrine, as in dropsical blood, or in the presence of certain substances which prevent coagulation: that place among which applies to carbonic acid." I know too that quantities of bloody fluid have been found in the chest where death has been perfectly natural. The fluid may have been there for some time before death and the discolouration was most likely *post mortem*, or it may have taken place at the time of dying. I do not think the appearance caused by irritation of the bowel by poison would be different to that caused by the irritation of natural disease. To the existence eight months after death of the grey mucous spoken of I should attach no importance. The practice for judicial purposes is to take notes at the *post mortem* at the time or soon afterwards. If there had been any marked ulceration, that might have been discovered after death by a careful examination of the interior of the bowel. Where there is waste from the body thirst is an occasional symptom. A person taking a large quantity of alcohol would experience thirst. I heard Dr Macintyre's description of the medicines he had prescribed. One of those contained opium and morphia, but the quantity was too small to have any marked effect. The depressing action of antimony depends upon the quantity. Very small quantities depress, and larger quantities increase the depression. In acute disease there is a greater tolerance of antimony. It is possible there may be a greater tolerance of antimony in some individuals than

in others; but I have had no experience of it. Without data as to the dose and frequency of administration I should hesitate to give an opinion as to whether death had been accelerated.

Cross-examined by Mr Haggitt: In cases of high fever and cerebral excitement patients can tolerate antimony. Uremic poisoning is not a very uncommon occurrence in Bright's disease and in kidney diseases. It is quite possible a man may have an incurable disease of a wasting character and yet die from some other cause. If there is disease of the heart the action of antimony would be more depressing than in another case; it would further depress the heart. Where there is debility from any cause the action of antimony would be to increase the debility. Antimony is not a drug that would be used for aged persons. In minute doses it might be given to aged persons if they were vigorous. I agree generally with the opinion that antimony should not be administered even medicinally to old people. The symptoms of antimonial poisoning are great depression, feeble heart action, profuse perspiration, vomiting and purging. Pain is also sometimes present.

Mr Haggitt: If in Captain Cain's case there were vomiting, diarrhœa, depression, frequent pulse, thirst and gradually increasing weakness, were they signs of antimonial poisoning?—I am to understand "if that were the case?"—because the pulse is described by one medical witness as very full.

His Honor: Where is the evidence of depression?

Mr Haggitt replied that Dr Macintyre had given evidence of the depression.

His Honor said the witness might have used the word depression in the sense of lowering the vital powers; but he could be asked if he meant depression of spirits.

Cross-examination continued: Depressed action of the heart might be separate from depression of the nervous system, but they generally went together. The symptoms mentioned were not inconsistent with antimonial poisoning, and were all features of antimonial poisoning. We do not necessarily expect to find all the symptoms in a case of poisoning. The most prominent symptoms in antimonial poisoning would be vomiting, diarrhœa, depression of the heart's action, and profuse perspiration. In this case if vomiting, diarrhœa, and depression of the heart's action were present, there were three out of the four most usual symptoms. If antimony was found in his body I should have no doubt it had been administered during life, and the antimony might account for the symptoms exhibited; but it would not absolutely necessarily follow that that was so if the deceased had not been in good health, but that would be a fair inference. If a person from natural causes exhibited such symptoms as sickness, diarrhœa, depression of the heart's action, and so on, the effect of administering antimony to him would be to depress him still further. Those symptoms would cause exhaustion and possibly death, and if antimony were given it would necessarily increase the other causes, and if given continuously it would bring about a fatal result more rapidly. One large dose of antimony might cause death. If on investigation I found one thing that would certainly cause sickness I should attribute it to the prominent cause, but that would not exclude my giving consideration to other causes which were possibly present.

Witness continued: The inflammation and irritation of the bowels might be produced by antimony. In seeking the cause of sickness one would have to go back further and seek the cause of the irritation. Antimony would be a sufficient cause for the symptom. I do not think simple effusion in the pleura would occasion cough. I do not agree with the opinion that blood may be expected to be found in the pleural cavity in every case of slow death. Disease of the heart would account for the cough though there was no actual disease of the lungs. In Bright's disease we generally find the body much wasted, but dropsy would mask it considerably. An examination of the brain might have shown whether there had been hemorrhage, notwithstanding that the body had been buried for eight months.

To Mr Chapman: When uremic poisoning follows upon Bright's disease it is a death by poisoning; the wasting process has not proceeded to its utmost length. The finding of fat under the skin is inconsistent with death from exhaustion by disease. It is quite possible for disease of the kidneys to terminate in uremic poisoning independently of the reception of any noxious substance. The last answer also applies to termination of life by apoplexy. A searching post mortem examination is the only certain means of distinguishing between those deaths, though the symptoms are sufficiently distinctive to enable a medical man to decide upon the cause of death if he has attended the patient. When I gave the answer that antimony would be a sufficient cause for the symptoms described, I meant if antimony were given in poisonous quantities, not necessarily large quantities. Medicinal doses occasionally produce what may be called poisonous symptoms, but not necessarily, as it is given in such minute quantities. Antimony is not a drug given to old people. I have no knowledge of the action of antimony on the spirits, but its action on the body is very marked. Depression of the body would in most people tend to produce depression of spirits. Sweating is one of the marked features produced by antimony. I am not at all surprised to find that Dr Macintyre in another case noticed the symptoms, and was struck by them. Dr Drew's description of the patient's pulse was that it was a full pulse, and that did not indicate depression. The talkativeness of the patient at that time did not indicate depression.

His Honor: Fat under the skin you said was inconsistent with death from exhaustion by disease, but it may be consistent with death from other causes?—Yes, your Honor. Assuming that some other cause than disease occasioned exhaustion, the exhaustion might be so rapid that the fatty tissue is not absorbed.

That would not be the case in an ordinary wasting disease which ran its course?—No; there you would expect to find little or no fat.

You instance uremic poisoning as a case which might occur and prove fatal, and prevent the disease from running its course?—Precisely. Of course the same remark applies to death by antimony, or any other poison?—Yes; or any intervening cause, such as inflammation of a vital organ, which might prove fatal in a few days. Then the death would not be from the exhaustion of disease.

In a chronic case like Cain's, would uremic poisoning develop itself suddenly so as to prove fatal?—The more common form of uremic poisoning is chronic; it comes on imperceptibly and slowly.

I would take your opinion to be this: that if uremic poisoning did exist, it is reasonable to suppose that it had been of considerable standing?—No; I meant by slowly, that it would come on in course of a few days or a few hours.

Were there symptoms of rapid uremic poisoning in Cain's case?—The symptoms of rapid uremic poisoning are striking; there were no symptoms of rapid uremic poisoning in this case.

Do the symptoms suggest anything to you—you can take them now in conjunction with the admitted appearance of the aorta and with the antimony found after death—what upon the whole do they suggest to you?—They suggest rather death by the lungs not acting.

That is caused by the imperfect oxydisation of the blood?—Yes.

That is caused by the weak heart action?—The weak heart action tends to produce that, and the diseased heart action more so.

Mr Haggitt: Would your Honor ask whether in rapid uremic poisoning there is not an entire suppression of the urine?

His Honor: Dr Alexander says in this case there is no symptom of rapid uremic poisoning.

Mr Chapman: No; nor did we ever suggest it, your Honor.

H. W. Maunsell, M.D., deposed: I have been over nine years in Dunedin, and was engaged in the practice of my profession for about 10 years previously. I heard Dr Macintyre describe the features of Captain Cain's case and the symptoms exhibited by Captain Cain the last time he saw him. I also heard the description given as to the manner of Cain's death. The condition in which Stubbs says he found him early in the morning may have been a condition of coma, and would be consistent with a natural result of Bright's disease. It may have been from uremic poisoning, or from the effusion of blood or serum on the brain. Old men with Bright's disease and diseased arteries frequently die of apoplexy. That is the kind of apoplexy described as extravasation of blood upon the brain. I have seen a large number of such cases. It is not at all a rare thing. Serous effusion upon the brain is also a common termination of Bright's disease. You may have effusion of any of the serous membranes of the body, and amongst others the brain. That causes pressure, drowsiness, and ultimate insensibility. Apoplexy in old people is also a recognised termination of Bright's disease. I have seen such cases; a few quite recently. There may be several attacks of effusion of blood on the brain. It may be sudden or it may extend over some hours. It would depend on the amount of extravasation of blood and the size of the bloodvessels that had given way.

In what part of the brain does the blood accumulate?—In any part where there are bloodvessels.

You have heard the symptoms accompanying Cain's death : are they consistent with either of these terminations of Bright's disease?—I think so. I heard most of Dr Ogston's examination, and I have had experience in a good number of *post mortems*.

In the case of a body in the condition described by Drs Macintyre and Hogg, having before you the symptoms described, do you think it would be practicable to make an examination of the brain?—I should most decidedly have had a look at the brain, with the fair hope of getting some result, or at any rate of determining whether I could get any result or not.

Supposing there were a clot of blood in the brain?—If it was a pretty large clot you might probably find it some months after death.

In *post mortems* what course do you follow, supposing you wish to examine the kidneys for Bright's disease?—I examine them microscopically or hand them to some pathologist to examine for me. If I had cause to suspect Bright's disease, and I had to examine a body even eight months after death, I should examine the kidneys if fair sections could be got.

Dr Hogg said he made sections of the liver : do you think, therefore, sections could be got of the kidneys?—Not necessarily so, but it might be tried. I think no organs should be left out.

Considerable importance was attributed by Dr Ogston to the absence of clots of blood from the heart; do you attach much importance to that?—No ; I do not think so.

Is it a circumstance tending to negative a natural death from disease?—No.

Then fluidity of blood has also been stated to be found in the cavity of the lung ; what would you infer from that?—You may have a fluid in the lung cavity due to something else than blood which may be only stained red. If I found that eight months after death, it would, if large, have probably occurred before death and be due to dropsy.

Supposing you were seeking exhaustively for the cause of death, do you think you could do so effectively if told there was vomiting and purging, without examining the whole of the intestinal canal?—I myself should examine the whole of the intestinal canal—split the whole thing from end to end.

Could you say whether any irritation would be due to poisoning or to gastro-enteritis?—I hardly think there would be any distinct difference between the two causes. I know the work of Woodman and Tidy. It is recognised as one of the best forensic works on medicine. I agree with the directions there given for the conduct of *post mortems*. The object of a *post mortem* is to ascertain the cause of death, and I should make it as exhaustive as possible. I think notes should be taken at the time which may be revised afterwards.

A thorough *post mortem* is an affair of three or four hours.

And in a case which may result in a serious charge you would not stint your time, care, or comfort?—No. I have a fair memory, but in a long and exhaustive examination I should not abandon notes and trust to my memory for three or four months.

We have heard of the Scotch and English practice, and I suppose I may add the Bohemian and Irish practice in such matters; is there any idfference in the way medical jurists do their work?—I do not think so. Notes to be of any value must be taken at the time. I think the instructions given in that book ought to be carried out. In all cases of this kind the object of a *post mortem* is to arrive at an accurate determination as to the cause of death.

Looking at the symptoms described by Dr Macintyre and at the results of the analysis described by Dr Black, do you consider that complete means were taken to determine the cause of death?—I could not state in such a case with absolute certainty what was the cause of death.

Do you think all means were exhausted, seeing that the head was not opened and the kidneys were not microscopically examined?—I think it would have been advisable to open the head.

Looking at the smallness of the quantity of antimony found by Dr Black, do you think it possible to say conclusively whether in this case antimony accelerated death?—You could not state with absolute certainty. It would be necessary as a factor to obtain some evidence as to when antimony was last administered. I think in Cain's condition antimony, if recently administered, would have done him a great deal of harm, even in small doses. I do not think it would be possible for a medical man to state positively that it accelerated death. It would be necessary to know the time of administration, doses, and so on. I heard Dr Alexander's evidence as to uremic poisoning and the termination of Bright's disease by apoplexy, and I think such a termination might have come on independently of antimony. I know the book of Woodman and Tidy. I approve of the cautions given there for conducting *post mortem* examinations. It would be necessary to keep the organs separate in order to get correct results in the different parts of the body. In connection with the determination of the administration, whether in one dose or recently, it would be necessary, if possible, to trace the quantity in the different organs. I heard Dr Alexander's description of the mode of action of uremic poisoning, and agree with its correctness. The condition described by Dr Macintyre, and spoken to by the witnesses Stubbs and Kay, was consistent with death by uremic poisoning.

Mr Haggitt (cross-examining): Was it als consistent with death by antimonial poisoning?

Witness: Not immediately with that.

Will you state kindly in what respect the symptoms differed?—During the last part of his life there is no evidence of vomiting.

Then, in antimonial poisoning does vomiting always extend to the time of death?—Sometimes; not always. Then, also, he did not have a clammy, cold sweat.

Is that inconsistent with antimonial poisoning that he should go off into a state of coma and not rouse himself up and die ?—It seems to be more like uremic.

Is it inconsistent, Dr Maunsell, I ask you, with any death from exhaustion?—No; sometimes people die in an unconscious condition.

Are those the symptoms from every death by exhaustion ?—No ; sometimes patients remain conscious up to the time of death.

Are they the usual symptoms of death in an old man?—Yes, if the lungs give away, they often are.

Then, Dr Maunsell, would not anything that tended to increase depression facilitate the death by exhaustion ?—Most decidedly so.

Is antimony a great depressent, or is it not?—A great depressent.

If antimony was administered to a man, then, who was already in a depressed state—we will even go the length of saying dying from exhaustion—would not the administration of antimony accelerate his death?—Yes.

If a man died of uremic poisoning, you would not expect to find antimony on him as a result, would you?—No.

Or if he died of any form of Bright's disease, antimony would not be developed?—No.

Or dropsy either?—No.

There is no disease that would develop antimony, I suppose?—No.

If you find many of the symptoms of antimony poisoning present during life, and if after death you find on post mortem examination antimony to exist in the body, what conclusion would you arrive at?—That he had taken antimony.

You would not conclude that he had Bright's disease, I suppose?—No, unless I knew that he had it.

I suppose you would conclude, if he exhibited symptoms of antimony poisoning and you found antimony after death, that the cause of death was antimony, and not that he might possibly have Bright's disease?—If I knew that he was dying from dropsy and Bright's disease I would have my doubts.

Would you have your doubts if he had dropsy and Bright's disease, and you found antimony in his body not eliminated, whether the antimony accelerated his death?—If I was certain that he had taken the antimony recently I would say that it had accelerated his death.

As long as antimony remains in the body does it not continue to act as a depressent?—It depends upon what part of the body you find it in. As long as it continued to be found in the urine it would act as a depressent, and so long it would be an accelerating cause of death. Antimony, even in very small doses, has a depressing action on the heart; and if the subject has heart disease the depressing effect is so much greater. I heard Dr Ogston say he had been concerned in 500 cases of post mortem examination. I am not a specialist in that way.

Then any question as to post mortem examinations might be as well put to any other sensible person?—I do not think so. If you say anyone who has received a special training as a medical man I agree with you. My opinion on the matter

is simply worth as much as that of any other medical man with similar experience as myself. I think in making a chemical or post mortem examination it is usual to take notes. The necessity for notes does not depend on the power of the memory but custom. It is a matter of form. I think it is a good custom.

His Honor: I do not think it is worth while pursuing this point any further. The fact is that Dr Ogston did not take notes. He might have taken them. Perhaps it would have been better if he had at the time; but I understand that a few days after he did put down his observations. These notes were not forthcoming, and he relied on his memory.

Mr Chapman (re-examining): You said as long as antimony was found in the urine it would continue to act as a depressent. Supposing that the urine, bladder, kidneys, some blood from the cavity of the belly, and part of the small intestines were put together, could you say on finding antimony that it was attributable to the urine?—No, I do not think so. There is fatty matter in or about the intestine and about the kidney. In a cas of retention and absorption of the urine the liver is one of the first portions of the body it reaches. I should not describe it as one of the remotest parts of the body.

Supposing antimony is found in a body and you know the patient was suffering from diseases sufficient to produce death, can you express an opinion as a medical man as to the effect the antimony had unless informed of all the circumstances of the case, when administered, and the quantity?—I should say in all probability it would hasten his death, but not with absolute certainty. I would not be absolutely certain it was given in his last illness at all.

You would bear in mind the experiments Orfila made?—Yes.

To his Honor: Diarrhœa during the last month of life would have a tendency to eliminate any antimony that might have been administered; so would vomiting.

Robt. Hall Bakewell, doctor of medicine, of the Universities of St. Andrew's and New Zealand, said: I have been 32 or 33 years practising in this and the old country, the West Indies, and the Crimea. In former times I had extensive experience in the use of antimony in medicine—both tartar emetic and the antimonial powder. These things are very little used now. I myself do not use them in one case in a hundred where I used to. Tartar emetic is, I think, superseded to a great extent by aconite, which has the same effect of allaying feverish excitement without inducing the same vomiting, nausea, and purging. This, and clammy sweats, enfeebled heart action and pulse, are the chief symptoms of antimony. These were the results wherever given in what I should call medicinal doses—that is, when the full effect was aimed at In the hospital where I studied we used to mix tartar emetic with salts, and it was the routine dose in all cases where we wished to allay feverish excitement. Even in those doses it acted well enough; but it was such an unpleasant remedy. People do not like such remedies that produce constant vomiting and retching. I have given as much as two grains in two hours to a man over 60. It was an acute case of double pneumonia; and the man was bled as well. He recovered, and he never vomited the whole time. The word "depressent" is rather a new term to me. I do not know whether a depressent of nervous systems on the heart's action is meant. Antimony does enfeeble the heart's action. I have heard Dr Macintyre's description of Cain's case and the description of Stubbs and other witnesses. The sickness produced by tartar emetic comes on within about an hour after administration, and continues in the case of a large dose until the whole has been got rid of. The retching is very marked and unpleasant, not like many other emetics that are vomited up and done with. It could not be confused with the effort of a person coughing up phlegm. The primary object of a *post mortem* I take to be to discover the cause of death. I should certainly examine the brain as well as the other organs. In every medico-legal case I always examine the brain as a matter of routine.

Mr Chapman: Even after a considerable lapse of time?

Witness: If the body is in such a state that a *post mortem* is at all possible, every cavity of the body should be opened. I find on reference to Caspar that it is absolutely required by German law.

Is he an authority?—One of the very highest.

Supposing that death had arisen from a clot of blood on the brain, would it be discovered eight months after death?—I have never made an examination after such a time, but if the other organs were in such a state that you could determine their state during life you would find the clot. I should expect to find the brain quite a pulp, but a clot might remain as something foreign to the brain substance. The description of Cain's symptoms is consistent with and as far as the data go suggestive of a natural termination of Bright's disease, viz., coma by uremic poisoning. You might also of course have an apoplectic clot. But looking at the drowsy state of the patient the symptoms were mostly suggestive of uremic poisoning. That is the natural termination of Bright's disease in about one-third of the cases. In fact if the disease of the kidneys continues you must have uremic poisoning. It is very difficult to distinguish the coma caused by apoplexy and uremic poisoning. Of course you can in the latter case test the breath with spirits of salts.

From the description you have heard from Dr Macintyre of Cain's symptoms can you form any conclusion as to whether Bright's disease was present?—I never was asked to form an opinion on such imperfect data, because of course I should have examined the urine, but I can only say that the probability is that the disease was there. I should expect to find vomiting in that disease. During the last few months I have had a case just the same as Cain's—an undoubted case of Bright's disease, in which there was vomiting, diarrhœa, and cough. It was an old woman, and she had heart disease as well.

The case was very like this one, then?—Only that she got better and went out of the hospital.

Perhaps she did not get four bottles of champagne a day?—No; nor yet any whisky. She wanted some, though. I was struck by the remarkable similarity of symptoms when reading the evidence of this case in the lower court. She was under my care at the time.

From what you know of Cain's symptoms is it reasonably possible for a medical man to form a decided opinion as to the actual cause of death?—Well, I have formed a decided opinion, but I am not prepared to swear that it was the cause of death.

May I ask what that opinion is?—Well, my opinion is that death was caused by uremic poisoning accelerated by alcoholic poisoning.

Supposing there was uremic poisoning, would the action of the antimony be to accelerate death by this uremic poisoning?—No, it would not necessarily be; particularly in this case, where there was so much alcoholic stimulant given.

His Honor: You mean that the stimulant would neutralise the effect of the antimony?

Witness: The antimony would, to a certain extent, be antagonistic to the action of the stimulant. I should rather put it in that way. Antimony would not accelerate uremic poisoning; by older writers, in fact, tartar emetic is recommended as a remedy for this particular disease. At all events it was a fair subject of discussion in my early days whether tartar emetic should or should not be given for this particular disease. Suppose it to have been given, it would have no connection with uremic poisoning. I recognise the publication produced ("The Practitioner" for 1870.) It speaks of arseniate of antimony being used in a pulmonary disease where there were frequent attacks of asthma.

His Honor: What is arseniate of antimony?

Witness: I suppose it would be a compound of arsenic and antimony.

Mr Haggitt (cross-examining): You said you would in a *post mortem* examine the brain as a matter of routine. In what state would you expect to find it after eight months?

Witness: I should expect to find it a pulp—about the consistency of cream. I have seen it so after a body had been six weeks exposed in the open air. It would be absolutely impossible to distinguish anything in the brain as brains.

You have said the symptoms described are consistent with Bright's disease: do you seem to be consistent with anything else?—From such data as that you might almost formulate anything. The symptoms might be those of antimonial poisoning.

Then why do you come to the conclusion that it was uremic poisoning accelerated by alcoholic poisoning?—Because in all cases of antimonial poisoning I have never seen a fatal case, and I have given such large doses of tartar emetic that I cannot believe two grains were fatal to a man in Cain's condition.

Not to a man 70 years of age suffering from heart disease of such a character as Dr Macintyre described on the evening before?—He was cheerful and lively, and therefore I say that two grains of tartar emetic had not been administered, or were not enough to cause death.

But why do you eliminate antimony from consideration altogether and lay no stress on its being there?—Because the symptoms 24 hours before death as described do not agree with antimonial poisoning, and they do with uremic poisoning. Antimony in small doses has a very transient effect except when administered to the extent of ulcerating the bowels. If its administration were continued, the effect would continue of course. I am considering that the effect of tartar emetic must have ceased some time before the man was cheerful and lively. If you saw a man take as much as I have you would say so. If you took two grains every four hours you would not be cheerful, I am sure.

Mr Haggitt: Oh, it takes less than that to destroy my cheerfulness, I can assure you.

Witness: The sickness was precisely not the sickness of tartar emetic. I heard Kay describe it, and the difference was so marked. He said no sooner was anything in his stomach than it was out again. That is quite impossible with tartar emetic. Had it been tartar emetic it could not have acted in that way.

What kind of sickness is the sickness of uremic poisoning?—I do not know that I have actually seen anyone vomiting from uremic poisoning. I did not stand by the bed of the woman whom I have mentioned in Christchurch, or examine the vomit in that case.

Do you say from the evidence of Kay and Stubbs that antimony must be thrown out of consideration altogether?—Not entirely, because I think antimony given to a man who had taken so much stimulant as Cain would rather retard death. Because there is no doubt that that stimulant was the very worst thing that could have been given him. All are agreed that the administration of alcohol save in very exceptional cases is most injurious in Bright's disease. Therefore I think that in the case of a man who had got under the influence of alcohol as Cain had small doses of tartar emetic would rather retard death than otherwise.

You assume that it was Bright's disease?—Well, Dr Macintyre said there was kidney disease and dropsy, and that albumen had been found in the urine; if that is not Bright's disease, I do not know what is. In the certificate of death he put kidney disease first and dropsy second.

Then you do first assume that he had Bright's disease?—I assume that he had what he was certified to have.

Then you assume that he had uremic poisoning, which is not a necessary attendant?—You cannot have any advanced Bright's disease without uremic poisoning supervening. I agree that vomiting in Bright's disease is the result of uremic poisoning. I could not say how long uremic poisoning has been known to exist. The condition of the patient may improve. I should not like to swear that I have known vomiting from uremic poisoning extend over a month.

Then, returning to the same question, why do you eliminate antimony altogether from consideration?—Because, as I have said, the administration of small doses of tartar emetic would be rather beneficial to the man. That is my only reason, together with the small quantity of antimony found in the body.

Mr Haggitt: You have heard that Dr Macintyre did not administer to him antimony: why do you suppose that antimony has been administered in medicinal quantities and for medicinal purposes?—I never assumed that.

Are you justified in eliminating the element of antimony from consideration in this case, unless you assume it to have been administered by a medical man and in medical quantities?—I assume from the small quantity found that it was administered in minute doses. I do not assume that it was given by a medical man, nor in what form it was given. I simply assumed from the absence of the symptoms of antimonial poisoning immediately preceding death, and the small quantity discovered after death, that it had been given in small doses for some time before death; otherwise I think it would have been found in much larger quantities in the body.

Why do you attribute the sickness to uremic poisoning and not to tartar emetic?—I told you that the character of the vomit described in the night preceding death was such that it could not have been produced by tartar emetic, but I do not say there was not at some period of the illness vomiting produced by tartar emetic.

May not the stomach be reduced to such a state by the administration of tartar emetic that at a subsequent period innocuous substances might have been vomited?—Yes, but then you would have other symptoms as well. You are assuming a state of inflammation almost. The effect of tartar emetic is very transient. We had to give it every three or four hours to keep up the effect.

Do you still think you are justified in eliminating the question of antimony entirely from the consideration of the case and saying that death was sufficiently accounted for by uremic poisoning accelerated by alcoholic poisoning?—I have told you I did not entirely eliminate it, because I have told you it would have a beneficial action in counteracting the effect of the stimuli. In the quantity mentioned and under the circumstances given, as far as my judgment goes, it did not and could not accelerate death. That is all I can say.

Notwithstanding he had advanced disease of the heart, disease of the kidneys, and dropsy as well?—If you stimulate a weak, thin heart like that, with valvular disease, you will do far more harm than by giving tartar emetic.

Witness continued: I never said I would give tartar emetic in such a case. I would not give it. It depends upon the nature of the heart disease as to whether or not it would produce depression. Any inflammatory cause would increase the heart's action. Increase of the heart's action is often an indication of weakness.

Mr Haggitt: Antimony found under such circumstances is not to be taken into account at all?—If you go on in this way all night you would not shake my opinion. For the third time I must repeat that I have taken the antimony into account, and I think from the quantity found in the body that when stimulants were being given the dose would be rather beneficial than not.

To Mr Chapman: When I spoke of small doses of antimony being likely to have a beneficial effect upon a person in Cain's state, I spoke with reference only to the fact that alcohol had been administered to the patient in large quantities.

(Some court documents having reference to the friendly suit brought by the accused in connection with his wife's property were put in evidence.)

Mr Chapman inquired what course the court intended to pursue. He was prepared to go on at once with his address, but as the trial had lasted seven days it could hardly be expected that he could conclude his address at once.

His Honor suggested that Mr Chapman should commence his address, and that when he reached a convenient point to leave off the court should adjourn and the address be resumed in the morning, remarking that it was for Mr Chapman to do what he thought best in the interests of his client. If an adjournment was desired it could be taken at once.

Mr Chapman thanked his Honor for his consideration, and elected to begin his address at once.

Mr Chapman in addressing the jury for the prisoner said that in the discussion the jury had just heard his Honor had suggested that he (Mr Chapman) should study the convenience of his client and endeavour rather to do the best in his interests than to give weight to any other consideration. That suggestion he would ask the jury to bear in mind throughout the remarks he would make to them. After the long trial they had heard, extending over seven days, occupied almost exclusively in taking evidence, he would have occasion to claim their indulgence to a greater extent perhaps than he had ever had occasion to claim the indulgence of a jury or of any other audience. It must be apparent to them that, looking at the issues involved in the case and the consequences involved, the position which he occupied in addressing himself to the subject under investigation was one of peculiar responsibility. He had felt that responsibility very deeply throughout the conduct of the case. On no occasion during the course of his life had he ever felt himself under so great a weight of responsibility; and he thought they would understand that when he told them that though he had been for a considerable time engaged in the practice of his profession, and had undertaken cases of considerable magnitude — civil cases involving very large interests—and had not entered the twentieth year of what he might call his apprenticeship, he had never before been called upon to undertake the defence of a fellow creature in a case in which from its nature his life might be said to be in peril. His sense of responsibility also arose out of certain circumstances connected with and peculiar to this case, which presented exceedingly rare features, and was of a character seldom found in the annals of trials under English law. The sense of

difficulty in dealing with the case did not arise out of the inherent features of the case, but wholly out of circumstances exterior to the facts which had a bearing upon the two issues the jury would have to consider when they applied their minds to the solution of the case before them. These considerations placed him under a feeling of peculiar responsibility, because he could not rid his mind of the impression that circumstances referring to another case, and having no direct reference to the issues the jury would have under consideration, could scarcely fail to raise in their minds a certain amount of feeling—he would not call it prejudice—which would, perhaps, unless he was able to lay the whole matter before them with great force, to some extent embarrass them in the determination of the true issue they had to try. There were certain issues that would present themselves to their minds when they came to the solution of this case, and he could not too strongly impress upon them the character of those issues and their duty in approaching a solution of them. The Crown in the prosecution had undertaken to prove that the man who was in the dock was guilty of having killed and murdered Henry Cain on the 29th of January of last year. It must have been obvious to the jury, from the way the learned Crown prosecutor had opened the case and up to the present time, that the question of the guilt of the prisoner necessarily divided itself into two main branches, and no doubt his Honor would direct them to bear in mind those two questions. The two issues for their consideration were:—Firstly, Was it affirmatively proved, and so conclusively proved that in their deliverance they would be able to say upon their oaths that Henry Cain met his death by poison? The other issue was—and he would ask them to remember that though the solution of that first issue was momentous in this case, the solution of the issue which lay behind it was the real one to which they would have to give their close attention,—namely, If they were satisfied clearly beyond any reasonable doubt that Cain's death was caused by poison, then was that poison administered by the prisoner at the bar? The jury must have seen as the evidence progressed that what, notwithstanding the opening of the learned Crown prosecutor that there would be no difficulty in concluding that the deceased had died of poison, the Crown from beginning to end had felt the real stress of was the other question, which would have to be determined before they could enter upon the consideration of the acts of the prisoner at all—namely, the question whether Henry Cain had died of poison or not. Roughly speaking, the evidence in the case had divided itself into three or four bodies. There was a body of witnesses called the first day who dealt solely with the question of the acts of the prisoner in connection with this matter, the evidence being directed as to whether the prisoner had any motive for bringing about Cain's death. Then there was another group of evidence—the evidence of the of bulk the medical men. A large proportion of Dr Macintyre's evidence, and of the evidence of Dr Drew and other medical men,

60 ·

was directed wholly to the question (as to which the Crown must take upon itself the affirmative), whether Cain's death was clearly, distinctly, and most satisfactorily proved to have been occasioned by poison. Another group of evidence which bore to some extent upon both these questions was the evidence of those persons who were in the house or who from time to time visited Captain Cain, and they would remember that the bulk of that evidence was directed to the question which his learned friend had opened as one the jury would had no difficulty in determining—namely, the preliminary question of whether Captain Cain died by poison. The first question, which did not necessarily and directly concern the prisoner at all, as to whether Cain died by poison, was one which they would have to scan with the same exactness, nicety, and scrupulousness as the second question—whether the prisoner was guilty of the administration or not. In dealing with the case he felt himself oppressed with considerable difficulty in endeavouring to disentangle the evidence so as to clearly, distinctly, and conclusively show the true history of the deceased for the period referred to, and still greater difficulty in determining what the Crown really propose as the line of proof on which they intended to rely in asking the jury upon their oaths to say that Cain died of poison. This difficulty arose out of a variety of circumstances. They would probably remember that the history of the case as opened by the Crown was a tolerably simple one. They were told that from a certain period—he thought it was in November—Captain Cain's whisky began to make him sick, and that there was something remarkable in the sickness—something distinctly traceable to the poison; that when the whisky was given up and champagne was given, that too made him sick, and that ultimately the cough mixture produced the same results. It was put to the jury that up to a certain period certain liquors and drugs produced no evil symptoms, and that then the same liquors and drugs for a certain period produced clear, distinct, and marked symptoms, which his learned friend undertook to prove were symptoms of poisoning by tartar emetic. Now, as the case proceeded they must have observed this feature in its history, and it was this feature that rendered it exceedingly difficult for him to concentrate upon one point or in any definite manner the criticism which he had to offer upon the case—the case as most distinctly opened by the Crown had in no manner and in no shape been attempted to be proved, but the attempt had been made to prove it from a totally different aspect. In the course of the case his learned friend had found it more than once necessary to change the whole front and bearing of the evidence in order to make it fit in with surprises which had arisen in the course of the Crown's own evidence. He (the learned counsel) might have misinterpreted the endeavour of the Crown, but he could point out the course that had been taken as illustrating the difficulties under which counsel for the prisoner necessarily laboured. His learned friend Mr Denniston and himself

had put their heads together in the matter. They had scrupulously and carefully scanned the whole case from Mr Haggitt's opening to the close of the evidence last week, and had scrupulously endeavoured to find out in a few words what was the case for the Crown, because his learned friend Mr Haggitt had, he maintained, wholly departed from the case as stated in his opening, and shifted his ground from time to time. They had honestly tried to find out what was the case for the Crown, and if he (Mr Chapman) had to address them in popular language in a somewhat rambling fashion over this portion of the evidence, he could only assure them that the circumstance was due to the extreme difficulty Mr Denniston and himself had found in putting their finger definitely on what the Crown intended to rely upon as the steps in their proof. But although they had some difficulty in this portion of the case, he thought he should be able to show that with the concluding part they had no difficulty at all. Something had been said in this portion of the case about precedure, and he had a remark or two to make about legal procedure in connection with cases of this kind. He was told—he knew himself nothing about Scotch law—that in Scotland the rule in criminal cases was this: In every case, when the whole evidence was closed, the counsel for the Crown summed up to the jury, and the prisoner's counsel followed in his address. He ventured to put it to them that in a case of this kind this would be a salutary practice; because if he could hear his learned friend now address them, he could tell what he really relied on as his case and the proof of the steps in it, and could probably compress what he had to say into half the time that he should probably occupy. But the English procedure—he did not know whether Dr Ogston would call it a loose one—was that if the accused found it necessary or advisable to call evidence, the order of the concluding remarks was altered, and his counsel was obliged to proceed with his address to the jury at once, even under the difficulty of not knowing what kind of case the Crown intended to attempt to make out. And in craving earnestly their indulgence, he should ask them to supplement him in the consideration of that case, as he thought he was entitled to do, representing a man in the prisoner's position, and request them to try not merely to listen to what he had to say, but actually to give him something more like active mental assistance in case they should seem him, as it were, missing the ground that the Crown would perhaps rely on. It was not an ordinary case that had lasted a day or two, but the evidence had spread itself over an enormous period, and owing to its bulk it was difficult or impossible for a man to reasonably carry it in his memory at once. When the jury came to a solution of the question he should ask them whatever bearing this or that portion of the evidence might have, and whatever his shortcomings might be in missing its bearing, never to forget these two considerations: It was absolutely incumbent on the Crown to affirmatively prove without reasonable doubt whatever issue the law cast on them; and it was incumbent upon them (the jury) to come to the consideration of the matter solemnly pledged on their oaths not to deal with anything as proved because he possibly had passed it over, and not to consider it so until they could refer it to their consciences and say that without any doubt at all this or that point must be considered as concluded. He could not too strongly dwell on the burden of proof that lay upon the Crown. His Honor would tell them that they were not to deal in surmises and the balancing of probabilities, or to consider any issue proved against the prisoner until every other reasonable hypothesis was exhausted and they found themselves carried away by the evidence and compelled to conclude any such matter as proved. As far as he could make out, it was not suggested in this case that Captain Cain's death was actually caused by the direct administration of poison. In almost all poisoning cases such a difficulty was comparatively easily disposed of. If a man was supposed to have had a dose of strychnine and it was proved there was never any real difficulty in determining that it caused his death, or if he had a dose of prussic acid it acted instantly. Such things did not as a rule leave open the question as to how death was occasioned. So in cases of acute antimonial poisoning. In a case of that kind which created a prodigious sensation in England some 10 years ago—the case of Mr Bravo—it was treated as a matter beyond all doubt. A large dose of antimony was found in his body, and it was proved beyond all doubt that he died of antimonial poisoning and that nothing else contributed to his death. The present case was distinct from any such case as that, because it was not suggested by the Crown that death was really caused by antimonial poisoning. The suggestion was something like this : The Crown took the burden of proving that a man whom Dr Macintyre described as suffering from mortal illness, concerning whom he made up his mind six months before the death that he must die, had eventually succumbed, not to the natural progress of his illness, but to antimonial poisoning. Long before Dr Macintyre had talked about his death as certain and had communicated as much to the members of the family, so that it could not be for a moment suggested that it was a secret to them or to Hall that it was only a question of time when Captain Cain died of the diseases from which he was suffering. As the doctor put it, he progressed from bad to worse, the illness taking the exact course he had anticipated, and he gave a certificate of death in the most ordinary way. That being so, it was a matter of extreme importance to consider what case the Crown really did wish and intend to make. They would remember the simple propositions with which his learned friend opened. Nothing could be simpler. The one question they would never have to consider at all was that involved in the issue, the burden of which the Crown had undertaken — viz., to show that Cain died by poison. It virtually came to this : The Crown undertook to prove that this man, suffering from these diseases, received antimony administered by the prisoner, and that but for the reception of this antimony he must most certainly have been

alive at a later date. The evidence by which the Crown had laboured to prove that issue was, taking it in bulk and analysing it as the jury would have to do, exclusively the opinion of those medical men who had been called for the prosecution. Now there was a difference between jurymen and doctors. A doctor entered the witness box, and however unbiassed he might be, and however good his intentions, he was put there to give the jury his opinion. The value of that opinion varied in various circumstances. If he only answered a question as to whether a bullet through the head before death would kill a man, his reply would probably be accepted as disposing of the matter, and be rightly endorsed by the tribunal. But between this and the opinions they had heard during the last 5 or 6 days he ventured to say there was such an enormous difference that the two things could not be classed together. A medical man summarised his experience (which might be *nil*), his reading (which might be imperfect and might be recent and ill digested), and what he had heard or discussed with others. Often it was a matter to which he had only addressed himself quite recently, and he was brought there to deliver an opinion, which he (the learned counsel) ventured to put it, was not valuable according to the confidence with which it was expressed, but in an exactly inverse ratio; because when the jury came to consider their duty in solving the question they would bear in mind that they were not dealing with matters of opinion only, but with opinions aiding them to treat questions which must be decided by affirmative proof. These opinions might bear weight according to many circumstances and many considerations. A man might be very confident in the witness box, might have a very happy way of answering questions, in an apparently conclusive way, and he might have a peculiar way of answering to questions of a particular person, who might be very skilled in questioning, and so he would venture to say that dependence upon skilled witnesses was a matter in regard to which the jury should be very guarded, or they might give weight to evidence which it in no way deserved, and might be led to an utterly fallacious conclusion. This consideration brought him to this, the jury should not merely accept the conclusions of medical men that were put before them, applying them as distinct, clear, and unanswerable proofs, but must be satisfied upon their consciences that they were unanswerable, and that they applied beyond a doubt to the question which they had before them for elucidation. Many writers upon the subject of scientific evidence, many critics of scientific evidence had attempted by means of articles, text books, and so on, to price or appreciate the value of such evidence, so that persons who had to deal with it might know exactly how far to rely upon it; but he would venture to say that their safest guide in matters of this kind was not to rely upon a medical opinion unless they found it conclusively backed up by the actual facts They would be told that they had, in determining these momentous issues, to find them absolutely proved, and he would show them that when they came to apply the proofs to the issues they would find that they were asked to pass this point—this bridge, so to speak—in reliance exclusively upon the speculative opinions of medical men, and that really there were no facts which they could adduce to support. in the conclusive sense in which it should be supported, the inference which they had asked them to accept. He scarcely need do more to illustrate his argument than to put it to them that in the multitude of differences among medical men—differences in argument, differences in weight of argument, differences of opinion as to the importance they would attach to this, that, or the other circumstance—the jury would find themselves considerably embarrassed in selecting from among the witnesses of the Crown the one whose opinion they would follow. And he would venture to say that if they got themselves into a difficulty in attempting to determine whose opinion they would follow, the difficulty would be increased, for his Honor would tell them that not only must the opinions agree but they must be backed up by facts to this extent, that in accepting it as a body and on dissecting it they must be satisfied that it conclusively carried them over the difficulty the solution of which they had to approach. Now what were the factors they had before them for the elucidation of this question? In the first place, as he had pointed out, they hac a tolerably clear history of this old man for a good many months. They were asked in the opening to rely upon the fact that at one time Captain Cain was in good health, and that after the prisoner became reconciled to him he became sick and was systematically sick after that, and some connection was suggested between the prisoner's approach and the sickness exhibited by Cain. This reference to the prisoner brought him to the subject of the second issue, but it was also connected with this portion of the case. Here he would ask them to consider this: His learned friend had promised to prove to them that the sickness was present at one period; that it commenced suddenly and was present in a marked way. That part of the case had been directly and completely disposed of by the evidence. Dr Macintyre did not appear to have been called in very often, and this old man, who was a tolerably robust man, appeared to have got over an older illness; but the weakness and the features of that illness appeared to have been carried on, and the doctor did not attend Cain again until the month of June before he died. The evidence of the doctor had been supplemented by evidence which must, he thought, have placed it beyond a doubt that this sickness was not a sickness which had a marked commencement at any particular time, which had reference to the prisoner's opportunities. They would remember that Mrs Newton, the dead man's own stepdaughter, and Bridget Wren had given important evidence upon this point. He was sorry they had not had those witnesses in court, and he would ask for very great consideration for any portion of their evidence which was in favour of the prisoner, because it would have been an advantage to the accused to have had a

searching examination of both these witnesses, and to have got out the full story of the people who were the real companions of Captain Cain — the continuous inmates of his house. One of these witnesses spoke of the sickness as an old affair, and the other spoke of it a so as having taken place at a time antecedent to the date when Hall became reconciled to Captain Cain. Mrs Newton said at one point, " I cannot tell when the captain began to vomit, it was an old thing so far as I know." Then she said further, " I saw father sick soon after I returned to the house in November." Then Bridget Wren expressly said in her evidence that the vomiting commenced at a date antecedent to Hall's reconciliation with the captain. At the latest it was October—a time when most distinctly Hall was not on speaking terms with Captain Cain, and much less was he on the terms of comparative intimacy, which commenced apparently some time in December. There was comparatively little evidence as to when Hall commenced to see Captain Cain at Woodlands, but this much was certain; that at first there was not so much a reconciliation as a renewed acquaintance, that this continued for a little time, and that later on there was a recommencement of something like intimacy. The date of these occurrences could not be fixed; but he ventured to put it to the jury, looking at the course of the case and the extreme fuluess with which the evidence had been taken, that had those two witnesses been put in the box, his learned friend Mr Haggitt, with the exhaustive examination to which he had subjected witnesses, and with the short cross-examination which would have followed, would have got out a multitude of facts bearing upon the history of Captain Cain's illnesses, and he would venture to say that the casual mention of prior sickuesses read from the depositions would have been greatly multiplied, and it might have been shown that this sickness was both frequent and continuous before, though it continued to intensify as the course described by Dr Macintyre and Miss Houston proceeded— namely, that the condition of the old man was going from bad to worse. That evidence had, however, been supplemented, but it had only been by singular good fortune that they had been able to pick up the scraps of supplemental evidence—the undisputed and indisputable evidence of three witnesses. Firstly, there was Miss Morris, who had been Mrs Hall's bridesmaid, and who lived in the house from April till June. This witness had told them that at an early date, when the captain was in no sense on speaking terms with Hall, he was at least three times sick during her stay in the house, and had on other occasions to have a basin placed beside him, so that in the event of sudden sickness coming on he could relieve himself in a proper way. These were circumstances to which, in the absence of a full examination of Mrs Newton and Mrs Wren, he asked the jury to attach great importance. Then came the casual reference to sickness made by Edwards, who knew Captain Cain but was not particularly intimate with him. That witness told them that upon one of the very occasions upon which Denis Wren had driven him to town Captain Cain was suddenly overcome with sickness in Slater's shop, and that he had not time to get out into the back yard but was overcome in the shop. The opportunities of the defence had been few, but the jury would observe that two persons had voluntarily come forward to state the fact of Cain's sickness at times when there could be no suggestion of it being from other than natural causes, and he asked them to supplement this by what they might be quite sure had been observed by other people. Up to the time that Dr Macintyre's attention was pointedly directed to sickness the old man did not probably think it worth while to tell the doctor about it. Until he got positively laid by, a sturdy old sailor like Captain Cain would have a positive dislike to complain to a doctor about minor ailments. Miss Houston said that she had heard of it, and so when the sickness actually occurred it did not present itself to her as a striking circumstance. Enormous importance had been attached to Cain's saying that it was a singular thing that he could not take whisky now—that it made him sick, although he had taken it for 50 years. Special importance had been attached to this because at that period of the case the Crown were going to prove that it was whisky which Cain drank, and that the poisoner had ascertained this fact and commenced to insert poison into his whisky. It was singular that sometimes in a case of this kind a momentous issue might depend upon a trifling thing. Whisky was used at the opening and all through the case until the examination of Mason came. The jury would remember that this witness was a vigorous young man, who, seemingly, was amused with this old gentleman, and was in the habit of sitting with him. He did say at first that Cain had told him whisky made him sick, but afterwards he corrected himself and said the expression the captain used was " grog." Seeing that Cain was in the habit of talking of whisky as whisky, not as grog, he put it to the jury as a fair inference that the old man's stomach had got into such a state that grog no longer agreed with him. Dr Macintyre described him as then in a hopeless illness, and was it singular that grog should disagree with him? As a matter of common experience some men could continue taking it to the end of their lives, others had to be very cautious, and others had finally to leave it off altogether. Moreover, when Mason came to tax his memory, he thought this took place early in November, and he did not understand the Crown to say that poisoning had commenced at this time. He ventured to put it that these circumstances were very strong and must have the greatest weight.

His Honor: It is on November 3, I think, that there is evidence of Dr Macintyre prescribing an effervescing mixture which he said was probably to relieve sickness.

Mr Chapman assented. The captain had so far given in then to the sickness. He did not think it worth while to tell the doctor of his actual vomitings, but at this date he told him he felt sick, and the doctor prescribed for him in order to ward off his sickness. He asked the jury to attach the greatest importance to this circumstance, as showing that the doctor had not a full and detailed history of the case. He now came to more nearly deal with the circumstances actually affecting the history of the case from the time it became more marked, and if he dealt with it somewhat diffusely he must again crave indulgence, seeing that even at that hour he could not put his finger upon the case for the Crown. Up to this point in the Crown's evidence there was a sudden break from health to vomiting, and the very moment was pointed out from which they might suppose poisoning commenced. Then later, the 24th December was taken up, and it was proposed to make that the starting point seemingly; and then the still later date at which Cain went finally to his bedroom was taken up. A singular feature about the evidence in support of slow poisoning was this: Whereas there was all kind of evidence as to sickness at different times, when his learned friend came to the medical evidence he entirely shifted his ground and asked the jury to found their verdict upon the medical evidence that poison was being administered exclusively during the last 14 days of Cain's life. Dr Macintyre was examined mainly upon the facts of the case, and partly upon the scientific features; Dr Drew mainly upon the scientific features and partly upon the facts; and the whole of the other medical witnesses were examined as scientists. The inferences to be drawn from the antecedent facts were confined by his learned friend to the fact of the administration of poison during the last 14 days of Cain's life. So the case necessarily stood thus. Supposing something were to crop up by some extraordinary process which he could not foresee, and the administration were clearly proved at that lunch spoken of by Mrs Ostler and Mrs Newton, the next question they would have to address themselves to was whether that poison administered at that time was proved to have accelerated death. And they would find that they had no evidence at all upon the subject. He was assuming that this was the state of facts at the time of the lunch and that it then ceased. So far from being possessed of any evidence on the point, the jury were deprived of any because his learned friend carefully shaped the whole of his questions to the medical gentlemen, not as to the effect of administering poison at various times spread over Cain's illness. To not one single witness was any other question put than as to the effect of poison if administered during the last 14 days of Cain's life. They were asked to pass their opinion solely and exclusively upon the assumption that poison had been administered during the last 14 days of Cain's life, and by inference they were asked to leave out of consideration any administration prior to that date; so that if it were now to appear conclusive to the minds of the jury that poison had been administered during that earlier period, or rather that it had been received during that earlier period, the scientific evidence in the case would give them no aid whatever. He did not know whether his learned friend saw the difficulty, but he could not credit him with having accidentally omitted to ask questions referring to the former period, and he had to assume that for some reason which was still obscure to him the learned counsel for the Crown had deliberately confined himself to the latter to the exclusion of the antecedent period. For some reason, however, which was to him inscrutable the counsel for the Crown at the twelvth hour —nay, at the last hour of the seventh day—began to ask Dr Bakewell, the last witness the defence had put in the box, what would be the effect of administering small doses of poison at a period extending prior to those 14 days—during the last month of Captain Cain's life. As to the exceedingly small quantity of anti-mony found in Captain Cain's body, he would ask them to say there was not the slightest evidence when it was received, because there was absolutely nothing that could satisfy their consciences as to when it was received. He did not wish to labour this point any further at present, but he had given them the key to what he meant. His learned friend had pinned his scientific evidence exclusively to the last 15 days or the last fortnight of Cain's life, and they must bear this in mind when they came to consider the question of motive as affecting the prisoner's acts and intentio is; and throughout they should never divest their minds of this, that the case became more and more unlikely the more they supposed the poisoner must have been satisfied that the man was a dying man from natural causes. He should presently put it to the jury, when he came to illustrate the true character of the evidence, as absolutely inconceivable—adopting his learned friend's chronology, the last 14 days to which alone the medical evidence had been addressed—that the prisoner should have proceeded, for the paltry considerations which he would show were the most he could expect to get out of the transaction, to cruelly kill a dying man. When he came to deal with the alleged motive he would satisfy them abundantly, he thought, that the motive suggested was perfectly ludicrous and must be swept to the winds. But in reference to the chronology of the case it seemed to him a singular and extra-ordinary thing that his learned friend should not have adduced a scrap of evidence as to the effect of the administration of small doses of antimony at an earlier period of Cain's sickness. He (the learned counsel) did not mean that they were to assume from anything he had said that he suggested that it had been administered at an earlier period of the sickness, but he was entitled to put it to them as strongly as this: Supposing they came to the conclusion that at one time the man had a sufficient motive for destroying a man who was not obviously in a dying state: and supposing they went so far as to assume that during that earlier period he actually did administer some poison, a poison which was said to have the effect in certain illnesses of accelerating death, they had now before them nothing to assist their judgment in coming to a conclusion as to whether it did accelerate his death. As a mere hypothesis he put this inference in the strongest

way against the man whom he was defending; and he put it to them that supposing they could from any antecedent belief as to the wicked-ness of the man come to the conclusion that he had done something at an earlier date—some-thing which it was said would do comparatively little harm or no harm to a healthy person—before they could come to the conclusion upon their oaths that that had accelerated death they would have to have testimony that it had accele-rated death; and yet, as he had pointed out, his learned friend had purposely left them bare of testimony upon that point. He put these facts and circumstances to them partly as illustrating the difficulty he was under in discussing this case, because he was probably breaking his teeth upon matters which his learned friend had virtually by this time abandoned, but as he had not the advantage of first hearing how the case was presented by the Crown he had to be careful not to omit any-thing which might be brought out when he would no longer be in a position to give them what he felt it to be his duty to give them—a certain amount of aid in coming to a con-clusion. For this reason he had to put the strongest presumptions against himself, and he would put it to them that his learned friend had by his medical evidence given them no aid in coming to a conclusion upon the subject. The counsel for the Crown had put the screw on the medical witnesses—the new-made medical ex-perts and the special expert,—and had almost succeeded in screwing them up to the sticking point and making them dogmatic—almost persuaded them that they could really tell that antimony must under certain circum-stances accelerate death. But giving the utmost weight to this evidence, to the strongest expressions his learned friend's ex-perience and ingenuity could drag out of his witnesses, he would venture to put it to the jury that that evidence only attempted to illustrate the case by reference to the effect of antimony administered during the last 14 days of a man's life. That part of the case he could safely leave, unless, owing to the long period of time the hearing of the case had covered, he had been mistaken in his recollection as to what questions his learned friend really did put to the scientific witnesses, and he would take the opportunity of seeing if he could have been in any way mistaken upon this point. The next matter for consideration would probably take him a considerable time, and he would therefore ask his Honor if this would be a convenient time for the adjourn-ment.

His Honor concurred in the suggestion that the court should adjourn, and the court adjourned at 6 p.m.

TUESDAY, FEBRUARY 1.

EIGHTH DAY OF THE TRIAL.

Mr Chapman (continuing his address for the defence) said the jury could not too strongly impress upon themselves that it was incum-bent upon the Crown to prove the case against the prisoner so completely and so affirmatively that they would inevitably be drawn to the conclusion that there was no escape from the reference of the prisoner's guilt. It was not sufficient, supposing, for instance, that there were ten possible hypotheses put before them and the Crown had succeeded in negativing nine of them. If there was one possible hypothesis which afforded sufficient, or apparently sufficient explanation of the circumstances which were laid before them, then they could not say that the issue the Crown had taken upon itself was conclusively proved. It was not incumbent upon the defence at all to explain the cause of death: it was the duty of the Crown to explain it in such a way that the evidence left them no possibility of drawing any inference other than that of the prisoner's guilt. As advocate for the accused it was his (the learned counsel's) duty to make suggestions to them consistent, or possibly consistent, with the evidence, or consistent with any reasonable inference to be drawn from it, so as to, as it were, stimulate the reasoning powers of the jury, and enable them to ventilate the subject fully. For the defence but a small amount of evidence had been called, and it had been called not to take up the burden of showing the cause of death, but to illustrate the succession of possibilities—indeed, of the strong probabilities—which would enable them to discover a natural explanation of the cause of death. One suggestion was that the natural mode of death in a case of the kind was death from uremic poisoning. It must have been pretty apparent to the jury that Cain had been suffering from Bright's disease. It was not necessary for the defence to show that conclusively, because they had it in evidence that any disease that paralysed the kidneys would cause an accumulation of urema, which finding its way to the brain would lead to the coma described in the evidence. Had the *post mortem* examination been really a complete one, and had it been conducted with a view to discovering the cause of death, something more definite might have been placed before the jury. It might be the case that microscopic examination of the kidneys would not clear up anything, but all the more prudent medical men, had said that it should have been attempted. There had been a good deal of apparent difference of opinion expressed by the medical men but very likely that was due to varying definitions; but it must have become perfectly clear to the jury that once it was established that Captain Cain had suffered from some form of Bright's disease there was an equally strong probability that it would terminate in uremic poisoning. Then there was another suggestion strongly insisted upon by some of the witnesses, that a disease of the kind from which Cain was apparently suffering very often had a sudden termination in consequence of a small artery giving way, and that was more usually the case where it was found that the arteries throughout the body were in a diseased state. Several gentlemen had told them that that was no uncommon thing; and Dr Maunsell had told them that he had had an instance of the kind in his practice recently, and that the mode in which

life terminated was through some small blood-vessel of the brain giving way. That was not spoken of as abnormal, and the same thing was spoken of by Dr Alexander and Dr Bakewell. There were thus three distinct modes in which life might terminate in a case of Bright's disease; and there was a further explanation offered by Dr Alexander, and again by Dr Bakewell, which was equally consented with the facts of the case as known. Dr Bakewell had said that the strong probability was that the excessive stimulation of which they had heard might of itself have actually brought about the state of coma. They had heard too from Dr Alexander that the common mode of the termination of life in these cases was entirely consistent with what Dr Ogston found—namely, a quantity of red fluid in the pleural cavities, insufficient aeration of blood in the lungs, leading to an accumulation of bad blood, through the blood being poisoned by carbonic acid gas through the insufficient action of air upon it. It was not his (Mr Chapman's) duty as an advocate to suggest these things, or in any way to prove them; but once they were seen as probabilities or as possibilites, he would venture to say that the Crown was precluded from saying that the cause of death had been conclusively proved to be such as the Crown took upon itself to prove against the prisoner. They must bear in mind in dealing with the case that it was not suggested that Cain died directly by antimony, but that death had been accelerated by antimony; and that it was in the plainest possible manner before them that even supposing that Cain had received antimony into his body within the time suggested by the Crown, all the various other causes of death might have operated perfectly independently of the contemporaneous action of antimony. During the case the jury had heard evidence as to the quantity of antimony which would produce definite effects, and that evidence must have left extremely vague impressions upon the jury. One great difficulty in investigating the matter had been to seize upon the time when it was suggested this antimony had been administered or taken, or to ascertain the quantity which was supposed to have been taken. He (the learned counsel) would ask them to bear in mind that Dr Bakewell had put it in this way, that supposing a small quantity of antimony had been received at a certain date, the action of the extreme doses of stimulants, as implied in the giving of four bottles of champagne in a day, would actually be neutralised by giving a small quantity of antimony. He did not suppose the jury would ignore the importance of that evidence, but supposing they did not attach much importance to it, that was only one of the possible explanations which he had been able to suggest, and it was here he would ask the jurors to supplement anything he had laid before them. It should not for a moment be forgotten that it was absolutely incumbent upon the Crown to prove that antimony was not merely received into Cain's body, but that it had been administered to Cain, and here a very large field opened up for suggesting innumerable possibilities as to how a small quantity of antimony might have been received. Dr Black's analysis disclosed the presence of about a quarter of a grain of tartar emetic, and by a rough calculation—he did not attribute slovenliness to the proceedings of Dr Black, for Dr Black had candidly said it was only a rough guess — it was estimated that there were in all about two grains of tartar emetic, of which only 36 per cent. was antimony. It would have been a matter of supreme importance in this case to have calculated not merely the quantity of antimony in the body, but a quantitative analysis showing the quantity presented by different parts of the body. That course was adopted in other cases, and should have been adopted here. Dr Ogston ha 1 had in this case an opportunity to distingnish himself as a t xicologist, and he would have done so had he investigated the case in a proper manner. It was true that a thorough investigation might not have led to more distinct results, but such an investigation should certainly have been undertaken. In a case of poisoning to which the learned counsel referred nine distinct parts had been taken up and kept in nine distinct jars, and the important turning point in that case was the various proportions found in the various parts of the body. The report showed that the various parts had been separately dealt with, and from this the authorities were able to draw important conclusions. Dr Ogston recognised the necessity for this in his evidence, for he said that he had taken four jars in such a manner as to illustrate reception, absorption, relention, and elimination, and the elimination was really the important thing in this investigation. Dr Maunsell had told them that had antimony been found in the urine in this case, as distinct from other parts of the body, it would have le1 him strongly to infer that antimony had been recently administered. But what had really been done? Dr Black had told them that the parts were mixed together. In the small vessel in which the urine was there were also the urinary bladder, the kidneys, some fluid scraped off from the cavity of the belly, or what was supposed to be fluid, and with the whole of these was actually mixed a part of the bowels a foot long. When he (the learned counsel) put it into Dr Ogston's hands, an authority which had been much used in the case, Woodman and Tidy's book, and showed him a quotation from Orfila, a high French authority upon the subject of the retention of antimony, the doctor had said it referred to the remoter parts of the body, but on reading it would be seen that antimony had been found in the fat, liver, and bones of a dog that had had antimony administered to it three and a-half months before death, and that similar results were obtained in a second case in which there had been an interval of four months. The liver was the first part of the body which antimony would reach after leaving the stomach, and fat was an element which was mixed in the jar with the urine. To put any of these parts into the same vessel with the urine entirely destroyed the effect of the supposed separation, because whatever was in one of these parts would be communicated

to the others, or at any rate the proportion would be destroyed, and anything that might be taken from the jar would represent not the separate contents of the various parts, but a mixture of the whole. This portion of the toxicologist's investigation had gone to the winds. Dr Ogston had told him his requirements, that he required to take something representing absorption, retention, and elimination separately, but when it came to be investigated it was found that though he had recognised his duty he had not done it. And what was the excuse? Firstly, that English customs were slipshod, and he had fallen into them. Then that he had only four bottles, and could not trust the Timaru bottles· and finally, that he had done a long day's work, or travelling, and that he was tired. He (the learned counsel) would tell the jury that Dr Ogston, with the supreme importance of the investigation necessarily in his mind, had wholly neglected his duty, which was to keep the parts separate in order to illustrate the true bearings of the case. There were a few criticisms which might be offered upon the whole subject of the manner in which the causes of Cain's death were sought by the gentleman who conducted the post mortem examination. It was conducted by Dr Ogston, a specialist and possibly the only gentleman in New Zealand who claimed to be a specialist on tne subject, though he would venture to say that many of our general practitioners had as good a title to the claim. Dr Hogg was also present, but in the presence of a man who claimed to be a specialist he would naturally take a subordinate part. The jury had had the slovenly manner of the post mortem pretty well illustrated, and he would venture to say that the proceedings of the post mortem were of such a character that they could not have met with the approval of Dr Hogg, a general practitioner in a country town. Counsel for the Crown had, not ventured to ask Dr Hogg for the mode in which this slovenly inquiry was conducted, and he (counsel for the defence) could not ask him because he had been put into the box before Dr Ogston; and he (the learned counsel) was not in possession of the astounding fact that the inquiry had been conducted in this lubberly fashion until Dr Ogston was cross-examined. He ventured to say that in the whole course of his practice he had never been more surprised than he was when by accident he tapped this line of the inquiry and found from Dr Ogston's own lips what had occurred. Even then he was not aware of the importance of the circumstances that a portion of the intestinal tract had been mixed with the urine, but he was filled with amazement in discovering the mode in which the investigation had been prosecuted. Dr Ogston had volunteered the statement that he had not proceeded to inquire into the causes of Cain's death, and that the main object of the inquiry was not to discover the cause of death, but to detect the presence of metallic poisons. Dr Ogston attempted to shelter himself behind the assertion as to his proceedings at this port mortem uy saying that though he had been brought up in Scotland, and apparently had reached middle life in the practice of his profession there, yet, on coming to an English colony, he had dropped into the loose English practice. The jurors happened to know that the place where Dr Ogston lived was Dunedin, and that Dunedin was not so very English that Scotch caution had departed from it. But there was really no difference between Scotch and English practice with regard to proceedings of this kind. In Scotland a medical man had to draw up a report within three or four days, and that report made on oath had a judicial value. In English courts no legal validity was given to such reports, but that was the whole difference in the practice, and there was no difference in any part of the world as to the mode of conducting a careful post mortem inquiry. What was Dr Ogston's explanation with regard to his making notes? He (Mr Chapman) would call attention to this circumstance, that the notes made by Dr Ogston during the trial had to be corrected in conference with Dr Hogg. Those notes were the substance of the Crown counsel's brief, and the witness was examined upon them for the first day; Dr Ogston then came to them the next day, and the counsel for the Crown intimated that he should ask a few more questions, and he did ask them. They now knew that the questions were asked after receiving from the witness a supplementary report. The proceedings of the previous day had jogged his memory, and he had given another report to be examined upon.

Mr Haggitt said that was an entire mistake. Dr Ogston had not given him a supplementary report.

Mr Chapman replied that it might have been that his learned friend had been coached verbally.

Mr Haggitt said he had only seen Dr Ogston for a few minutes.

Mr Chapman had no doubt that in those few minutes the coaching was done, and that the gentleman whose memory was so perfect that he might depend upon it at a distance of four months as so infallible that he might swear to appearances in Cain's body so confidently that a fellow-creature's life might depend upon the result—this gentleman whose memory was so perfect and trustworthy had actually to get the counsel for the Crown to examine him the second day upon alleged suspicious circumstances which were not examined upon during the first day. It was during the second examination that Dr Ogston was questioned on the subject of the fluidity of the blood and the quantity of blood in the pleural cavity, and the alleged suspicious aspect of these particular features. He would put it to the jury that from beginning to end there had been no true post mortem examination made or attempted. He had dealt only on one or two particular circumstances, but would venture to say there were a hundred things Dr Ogston had failed to investigate which he ought as a matter of duty to the State and his fellow men, to have investigated, in order that the true causes of Cain's death might not be left a matter of speculation. There had been a failure to examine the brain

in this case, and Dr Ogston had founded his justification for not examining it upon his experience in 500 cases, which, however, on cross-examination came to be be reduced to one baby and a man who was drowned. It was true that an examination of the brain might only have verified Dr Ogston's opinion; but it should have been verified; and they had the testimony of qualified persons that a great clot of blood in the head would have been apparent even when the brain had degenerated. The doctor did not examine the intestinal trachea beyond taking out a few small pieces. These matters he suggested to the consideration of the jury as showing that an examination never was properly made, and that they had not been put into possession of the results of anything like a reasonable investigation of the causes of Cain's death. Could they upon such evidence deal with the question which might possibly involve the life of a fellow creature? He ventured to think that if the life of the prisoner was at any time in peril during the course of the trial it ceased to be a peril when they heard Dr Ogston. They had been told by Dr Ogston that he determined to make no search for vegetable poisons because of the lapse of time after death. He (the learned counsel) attached little importance to that because the vegetable poisons atropia and colchicum had long since been abandoned on behalf of the Crown, though he (counsel) ventured to say, in view of the authorities which had been referred to, that it would have been a profitable thing to have searched for those poisons. Dr Ogston had told them that his investigation had not been so much into the causes of Cain's death as to trace antimonial poisoning. It would be idle to attempt to ignore the circumstances of the other case which had been given in evidence. Dr Ogston was one of the witnesses for the Crown in that case; and it was obvious from Dr Black's evidence that in the other case poison had been administered in enormous quantities. Starting from that point, Dr Ogston had evidently concluded that the sickness of Captain Cain must have been caused by antimony, and had approached the case with the absolute feeling of certainty that if he found antimony there he would find it in such quantities as completely to explain the whole thing at once. This explained the whole course of the slovenly proceedings and the expression that the main object was the search for antimony. He (counsel) had endeavoured to deal not fully but to some extent with the apparent and actual causes of Cain's death, but it must be understood that he did not accept the burden of showing of what Cain died. It was sufficient for his purpose to show that no endeavour had been made to demonstrate that the cause of death was inconsistent with any other explanation than that he had died by antimony. In a recorded case in which it was alleged that the death of a person suffering from a mortal disease had been accelerated by antimony, in which the evidence was as strong as in the case before them, the jury had no hesitation in throwing off the responsi-

68

bility of convicting, as there was a reasonable explanation of the death otherwise. Coming to the second issue of the case, he would say that, supposing by any process they came to the conclusion that Cain's death was appreciably accelerated by antimony, then the law cast upon the Crown to prove conclusively, so as to leave no other reasonable hypothesis, that the poison was administered by the prisoner Hall. He ventured to say that vague as the proofs were upon the other issue, they were more vague in this. A very little ingenuity would show the jury that others than the prisoner had an equally strong motive for desiring Cain's death, and that there were innumerable opportunities for them to carry out their desires. He wished it to be distinctly understood that he made no charges or imputations against anybody; he merely suggested possibilities. The counsel for the Crown would have to admit that under ordinary circumstances it would be preposterous to put a man upon his trial upon the evidence bearing upon this case. The Crown must rely upon impressions derived from another case, and he contended that it was utterly fallacious to trust to impressions from the other case, because there was not the barest trace of similarity between the symptoms existing in the cases. With regard to motive, they must consider the adequacy of motives, for no one could recognise as a motive something which was a wholly inadequate explanation of the actions proposed to be explained. The benefit to be derived by Hall under the settlements from Cain's death was very trifling; and inasmuch as Hall had not objected to his wife making a settlement, in conjunction with her sister, under which an annuity of £300 per annum was to be paid to Captain Cain, he must have known that Cain had not much to leave to his stepdaughters, and it was by no means certain that they would receive anything Hall, in December, agreed to this settlement, and was it to be supposed that he killed him the next month for some advantages supposed to come out of Cain's estate? The real reliance as to motive was upon the double settlement of 1870, and the settlement of Mrs Hall's own property, but the facts which had come out in evidence showed that reliance upon those settlements had absolutely gone to the wall. It had been conclusively shown that it was known to Hall that Cain was a dying man, and surely nothing could be more just, reasonable, or fair than that this annuity and house should be given to an old man who was virtually in a dying state. Dr Macintyre had told them that Cain could not live long; and were they to suppose that Hall put an end to this man to destroy an annuity which he had granted a few weeks before? Surely nothing could be more preposterous than that suggestion. The prisoner would gain no ready cash by Cain's death, and the motive suggested was that to save possibly three months of an annuity of £150, to get back £37 10s which the prisoner had but a few weeks before granted, he had killed an old and dying man. For that doubtful advantage it was suggested the prisoner had committed the crime. Then as to Mrs Hall's independent property, the motive suggested in connection with it also vanished into thin air on inspection. Through a conveyancing mistake Mrs Hall had settled her property upon herself, so that she could only dispose of it by will. The theory was that there was some sort of dispute about this, and that Hall wanted a suit in equity to set aside that particular provision which eliminated Mrs Hall's disposing power. It was suggested that Captain Cain, who was merely a trustee, would not consent to the alteration of the settlement, but the fact was that it could have been altered without his consent, and that he had consented to the alteration, as was shown by the affidavit of Cain, which had been put in evidence. Amongst all matters, the only one in which they could trace a fragment of pecuniary interest was the possibility of getting some old furniture, half interest in a bit of land, and the destruction of the annuity, which might have brought to the prisoner an advantage of from £30 to £40. The Crown must rely upon these as motives, but the jury had to look for adequacy of motive, and motive was only intelligible upon the assumption that the advantage to be reaped would get a man out of a pressing position. That being so, what possible aid could Hall derive from Cain's death? It had been put forward, they would remember, in the other painful case, that Hall had resorted to crime for the purpose of getting ready money enough to completely clear him from his difficulties. Now, whatever conceivable gain could be got by Cain's death, it could not yield ready money, but it yielded additional expense in putting Woodlands in order, and could not help the prisoner to get money to meet the forged bills. The biggest forgery which had been put in evidence was withdrawn and had been put out of sight. The forgeries with which the prisoner was oppressed were all small ones. Any one of them might have been met by a comparatively small cheque, and they had this salient fact, that in December and January—the period over which this poisoning was alleged to have been spread—Hall's private banking account was uniformly in credit to amounts varying from £300 to £500, and almost always in credit to the extent of £500; while the banker had told them that the prisoner would have no difficulty in overdrawing to the extent of £200. He (Mr Chapman) then went on to refer to the poisons which the Crown had proved to have been purchased by Hall. Now Hall had been engaged in photography, and there were at least three, and probably a dozen more, deadly poisons which might have been shown to have been in his possession. But that did not suit the prosecution. They started with one assumption, and everything was worked up to that. It was shown by Mr Wakefield's evidence that regarding the book Mr Hutton had been absolutely mistaken. But even supposing the book had been borrowed from Mr Hutton, it was not a book on poisons at all, but a book on the action of medicines, and it dealt with antimony as a medicine and not as a deadly poison.

Then it appeared that from the very first to the last Hall had no desire even to make the acquaintance of Captain Cain, and yet they were told, when this casually came about, that Hall set about some murderous design of destroying him. A great deal had been made out of Dr Ogston's evidence by the other side, and it appeared to be the prop, the pillar, and the stand-by of the whole concern. He had stated that unless a man wished to poison himself he would not use antimony in cigarettes in the manner suggested. Now, it was a most singular thing that on searching amongst authorities they had found that antimony had actually been used in this way in cases of asthma; and Gunn's evidence showed that he and Dr Lovegrove suggested methods by which it might be tried. If Hall had intended to kill Cain there was every likelihood that he would be very chary in what he did, but in all they had heard there was nothing to show that in what he did he could not have been readily observed. The table on which the medicines were kept was in full view of a window from the verandah; and Denis Wren had stated that anyone opening the door would surprise any person who was tampering with the medicines, so that the suggestion that the medicines had been poisoned was one involving a proceeding fraught with danger. Then there was no connection in point of time between Hall's visits and Cain's sickness; and though it was open to anyone to take these liquors, the only other instance of sickness was one or two trifling cases, which might easily have been caused by the smell in the sick room. Another point was that a special bottle of whisky had been set apart for the men. The only observation he had to make about that was that it never made the men sick, but it did actually make Captain Cain sick. Under these conditions almost anything would have made him sick, and the whole of this sickness was consistent with the explanation afterwards given by the doctor—that Cain was suffering from an illness that must prove fatal, and naturally produced sickness. Rum was tried by way of a change, and it made Cain sick. Brandy was tried on one occasion—taken quite accidentally,—and the moment the old gentleman got this brandy down his throat it was thrown up very much in the same way. Port wine, too, was given on one occasion as a surprise, and it too made the old man sick. He commented on the absence of Mrs Newton and Mrs Wren at this trial. Their absence, he knew, was due to circumstances for which he did not propose to hold the Crown responsible, but still it would have been better if they could have been cross-examined, so as to elicit something more about the history of this strange household, they being the only persons who had an intimate connection with the provisions, the food, the liquors, and their administration to the deceased. The mystery of the cupboard incident had been fully cleared up by Mrs Newton's evidence. Cain having refused whisky from the ordinary bottle which was on the table, somebody suggested that there was wine in the cupboard, and Hall being the only man present besides the invalid, it was only natural that he should have gone to the cupboard for it. This wine had made him sick, but it was taken at a time when he had taken to being sick. His learned friend's opening was so different from the grounds to which he had shifted that he hardly knew what he intended to rely upon in summing up. The Crown seemed to start with the assumption of the man's guilt, and everything had to be bent in that direction—including the slovenly post mortem examination ignoring all search for other poisons, or any search for the true cause of death. Cain was in the habit of travelling about, and he might have obtained medicines from Dunedin or Invercargill. They did not know his sources of supply, or indeed the sources of supply for other persons who were living in the house. They knew this much, that there was no want of familiarity with poisons among those in the house, because on one occasion the druggist told them of the purchase of as large a quantity as 1oz of strychnine. He said that against some of these people just as good a story might be weaved as against Hall; and yet they were all equally innocent. The persons who actually gave Cain medicines and drinks were innumerable. At this point his learned friend got into one of his difficulties. He brought in symptoms and references concerning this other case with the view of showing that this man was capable of such a thing, and so on. The only reference he (Mr Chapman) should make to the other case was this: The jury must remember that it was four or five months later, and they were not entitled to give any more weight to it than the law allowed to them to. If they tried to elucidate it they would find that the whole method in this case was different. There was no evidence as to how the antimony got there. If administered, it must have been by the most subtle means and in the smallest quantities, and the whole found was consistent with a single dose, and this result follows. The Crown were trying to show that antimony must have been administered to this old man shortly before his death, and yet the singular circumstance stood out more clearly than anything else that not a single scrap of evidence had been adduced to show that Hall on the 26th, 27th, and 28th—the three days before the death—was in the house at all. Yet the old man was said to have received antimony in his wines or medicines immediately before death. He submitted that this showed the supreme importance of a proper post mortem, and in not following the proper procedure Dr Ogston had gravely and grossly neglected his duty to his country and his fellow man. Though he did not wish to say anything unduly harsh of that gentleman, he would not shirk his duty, and would put it to them strongly that Dr Ogston had gravely neglected his duty both as to the extraction of these parts of the body and in the manner in which he had slummed the investigation and failed to take notes. In speaking of the colour that was given to the case vast importance was attached to small circumstances. A witness named Gardiner was brought all the way from Timaru to prove that Hall intended to take a house, but did not in view of Cain's approaching death. It must be remembered that Cain's condition was unknown at the time to Gardiner, and what impressed him was the news that his old acquaintance, whom he had recently seen about, was brought to such a pass. Then as to Hall's conversation with Miss Gillon in which he said it was a pity the doctors could not give Cain something to put him out of his misery, it was only in cross-examination he elicited the conclusion of Hall's sentence, "because he was struggling so." What Cain complained of from the beginning was his cough· and there was nothing singular or inhuman in an expression of the kind. Had not most of them heard it remarked in cases of the kind that it was a pity medical men had not authority to release a man from his suffering? In houses where people had died painfully such expressions were far from uncommon. And if Hall were poisoning the man he could not have made use of even this commonplace expression, seeing that it tended towards a sort of admission. They must remember that but for the shadow of the other case there would not be the slightest suspicion against this man. They were not to imagine that because he was suffering durance for one offence therefore he was guilty of another. If that line of reasoning were open, evidence would be beside the question. They had either to decide the case on the evidence against the prisoner or without regard to that evidence, and they were on their oaths to decide not without the evidence but scrupulously in accordance with it, and bearing in mind that the whole burden of proof rested with the Crown, not with the prisoner. And the case as it stood rested entirely on the mere opinions of medical men; the Crown could not screw out of any of them more than an expression of opinion, and when it came to placing absolute reliance on the opinion of a witness they must solemnly remember that their oaths did not allow them to let any man's opinion outweigh their own consciences and exclude or take the place of their own judgment. In cases of this kind there was always danger of a hasty conclusion, and they must treat it as having to be proved so carefully that it was carried beyond any reasonable doubt that the whole of the facts were inconsistent with any other rational conclusion. Such a verdict as "Not proven" in cases which presented suspicion only was not known to the English law, and if they found the proofs in any way fell short of completeness it would be their duty to return a verdict of "Not guilty." He ventured to say that the circumstances of the other case that had been referred to, though it might tell against the prisoner, would in a certain way relieve the minds of the jury, because it could not be put to the jury, as was sometimes done, that they were relieving themselves of responsibility by turning the man adrift among society. Here their verdict of acquittal would only have the effect of consigning this man to the punishment that had been awarded him by another tribunal.

He referred to this only because of the fear lest they should be induced to give too much weight to the circumstance that he had been convicted by another tribunal. The strongest evidence put before them was opinions, wherein medical men never ventured to say that antimony did accelerate the death, but only that it might. It was a singular thing, too, that the only man who had had experience of antimony— Dr Bakewell, perhaps the oldest medical man who was called—did not find the matter so formidable. There was extreme danger in trying to solve a problem guided only by outside opinion; and the learned counsel proceeded to quote various instances within the last 20 years of men having been unjustly convicted and sentenced. Capital cases had to be approached with the utmost caution; and in connection with the present case this had been instanced in the trial of a young lady for attempted murder, who had a day or two ago appeared in the witness box and given evidence. He must say he felt a certain relief and pleasure that that young lady should be allowed to stand in the witness box and tell her own story and clear herself, once for all, from the last fragments of suspicion that might attach to her. She was tried on a wholly mistaken apprehension of the case before the court, and he put this before them as an example of the extreme danger of drawing hasty inferences from inconclusive proofs. He had done his best both in the examination of witnesses and in endeavouring to put before them all the facts in favour of the prisoner, and he must acknowledge himself more deeply indebted than he could express to Mr Denniston for the way he had supplemented him throughout that long and anxious case. He had received from him every conceivable help, and if he had imperfectly represented the extreme doubt there was about the evidence and the danger of a hasty inference, it must be attributed not to the inherent weakness of the case but to the imperfections of his own advocacy. He felt satisfied he could now leave the matter safely in the hands of the jury. They had to determine questions which clearly involved the life of a fellow creature, and he felt confident they would use the utmost of their judgment in putting together the facts and looking at every aspect of the case to determine the issues now before them.

It being now 1.15 p.m., the luncheon adjournment was taken, after which

Mr Haggitt replied on behalf of the Crown. It was unnecessary for him to make such a speech as that of his learned friend; but he would confine himself to the three issues placed before them. Nothing could be more clearly proved than that the death of Captain Cain was due to poisoning. They had heard that even a two-grain dose would be sufficient to cause death, and the same would be the result if a succession of small doses was continued. The evidence conclusively established this fact: that whatever the state of Captain Cain might have been, whether he really suffered from kidney disease or Bright's disease or not, or whether he was dropsical or not, the tendency of antimony would be to produce a state of depression hat would result in death. It was not necessary that they should prove death was occasioned by it, but only accelerated. As regarded the next point, that antimony must have been administered to him during his life, the symptoms and the medical men agreed on this. The whole of the symptoms often did not occur, but those Cain exhibited during the latter period of his life were absolutely consistent with the fact of antimonial poisoning going on at the time; and they had this incontestable fact which his learned friend had not attempted to touch upon, that antimony was found in the body after exhumation, and the finding of that was conclusive of the fact that some or all of the symptoms of antimonial poisoning must have been present, and antimony even in small doses was sufficient to cause or accelerate death. All the medical witnesses were agreed upon this point with the one exception of Dr Bakewell, whom they could well afford to ignore. The jury had heard how he gave his evidence, fencing and evading direct replies, and he left that testimony in their hands. The symptoms continued down to the death, and there was positive evidence that even on the last night sickness and diarrhœa continued. The question next to consider was, How did the antimony get there? He submitted that upon the evidence the prisoner alone had the poison, and would, could, and might administer it. Everyone else who was about the captain had been called and examined. It was not likely that Cain would have poisoned himself—more especially with antimony which was an exhausting and lingering death. It was the last poison a man would make use of against himself, and there was the direct evidence of Mrs Ostler that he was anxious to live. It was so utterly unpleasant as to be impossible that a man should choose such a poison as tartar emetic, attended by such symptoms and causing death by slow exhaustion. So any theory of suicide was out of the question. They were then driven to a last resource, the administration by someone else. He had exhausted the subject of suicide and administration by anyone else, with the result that the only person left unaccounted for was the prisoner. What was there now that pointed to him? In the first place, it was a very unusual coincidence that he should have made the subject of poisoning a special study. That he did so was proved conclusively. A great deal had been done and said about Hutton's evidence, but really his evidence was not nearly so strong as that which the prisoner had called for himself. Hutton was not called to prove that Hal' falsified his entry in the cover of the book, and he failed to see what that had to do with the death of Cain, but his learned friend had tried to make out this as of the utmost importance. The jury must see for themselves that the only reason the evidence was introduced was that he had made it a special study. The evidence of Mr Wakefield, that he had the book sometime during 1884, and of Mr Hibbard, that he had it during the winter of 1884 or 1883, only went to increase the time over which the prisoner's opportunities of studying the subject extended. The Crown could only prove possession in May 1885, but his learned

friend had proved that two years before that time Hall had made the subject a special study. None of the witnesses said it was the same copy. They all might be right, and it was possible that Hall had given away his first copy, or it might still be in his possession undiscovered. First, then, he said that Hall had made poisoning a study, and next that he had poison in his possession. Had they not heard of the quantities of poisons purchased by the prisoner? On the 20th of March 1885 he bought atropia, and in May two drachms of tartar emetic equal to 120 grains, which if administered in two grain doses would make 60 doses in that one packet. There was, further, the circumstances of his borrowing the pestle and mortar and of his buying more atropia, &c. The medical men who gave evidence spoke to the effect that these poisons—colchicum and atropia—were not of a character to be traced, and they dropped out of the analysis; but the jury might still take into consideration that these poisons were in the prisoner's possession. There were two points thus established—first, the studying of poisons, and secondly, possession of poisons. The third point he would make was that the prisoner had opportunities of administering it. Of this the jury could have no doubt—he was there daily. Mr Chapman had said that there was no evidence of his being there on the 26th, 27th, or 28th January, but this was a mistake, for several witnesses saw the prisoner there on those days, and they had evidence that his visits were daily.

Mr Chapman: no one was examined as to those three days.

Mr Denniston: Yes; No one who was there during the last three days was asked one question as to whether they had seen Hall there.

Mr Haggitt said it would be strange if Hall was in the habit of going there every day, then dropped it suddenly, and turned up again at almost the moment of the death. There was evidence that he was actually there at the moment of death. It was no part of the prosecution's duty to show how the poison was administered; it was sufficient to show that he had an opportunity. His learned friend had twitted him with the case having been worked out differently from what was opened by the Crown, but in this he was again mistaken. The case that was opened was the case they had proved. They said that at one time the poison might have been administered in whisky; he did not say it was—it might have been contained in the glass, or the water mixed with the whisky. It might, on the other hand, have all been administered in the cough mixture, by which he had shown it was finally administered. He had given the jury first the case in which wine was administered and sickness afterwards resulted, but he did not pretend to say that it was the fatal case; and there had been no shifting of his ground. They said that his health was undermined by doses from time to time, and that finally his life was exhausted by small doses It was not possible to say on what day the dose was administered by the prisoner which proved fatal. The vehicle of the poison might have been altered a dozen times, for all the Crown knew. They simply said that the symptoms were there, and that the result had proved that antimony had been administered. It was for the jury to trace the cause and effect, and in doing so they must attribute the result to the antimony. It was not possible or necessary for the Crown to say the times and circumstances of the doses; that was a fact probably known to the prisoner and to no one else. He had no accomplices, nor were any necessary. Did the jury believe the prisoner carried a vial of tartar emetic in his pocket? If so, what could be easier than for him to drop it into the cough mixture after giving Cain a dose himself? No sickness would follow the dose he gave him, but every other one out of the bottle would produce nausea or sickness. Science told them that the antimony must have been administered by someone, and the most they could do was to point out the probabilities The next evidence was that the prisoner had a motive. The next circumstance pointing to the prisoner's guilt was that he had a motive for the commission of the crime. The learned counsel for the prisoner had said that the Crown had suggested motives for the offence, and had then failed to prove them. He did not think for a single moment that his learned friend was right in that contention, but maintained that the motive as indicated had been proved conclusively. It was, however, no part of the case for the Crown to suggest or to prove a motive. That element could be entirely left out of the case, and the jury need not trouble themselves as to what the prisoner's motives were if they were satisfied that he administered the poison. The prisoner might have been actuated by an entirely different motive from the one suggested—the Crown were not bound to suggest, or the jury to find the actual motive. It might be that the act was done from pure malice, or simply from dislike to Captain Cain. Such cases had been in which there had been no apparent motive. The Crown in this case suggested a pecuniary motive, and as there was evidence to point to the fact that such a motive did exist, it was quite right to bring the evidence forward; but it did not by any means follow that if they failed to prove the motive the case was weakened. In the mind of the prisoner there might perhaps have been no motive at all. Perhaps the desire, such as had been known to seize persons who dabbled in poisons, to kill simply for the sake of killing might have taken possession of the prisoner. The learned counsel for the prisoner had called attention to a number of cases wherein he said justice had gone wrong, and he (the learned Crown prosecutor) could call attention to a number of cases where death by poison had been caused without the slightest motive being attributable to the prisoner beyond the desire to destroy life. He thought it probable some of the jurors had noticed in the papers not long ago a case where a woman had poisoned 470 odd people just for the sake of poisoning them. When the idea of poisoning entered into the mind of a human being, and

when he saw the power that the possession of poison gave him to remove everybody that stood in his road; when he knew from a study of poisoning the difficulties that existed in tracing the means he had adopted—the almost absolute impossibility that existed in many cases of even tracing the poison that was used, it was not to be wondered at that when a man had reached a state at which he could resort to poisoning at all, that he would proceed in his poisoning without any adequate motive, or without any motive at all. So he would say to the jury, as a matter of law, that the Crown was not bound to prove or to suggest a motive, but he asserted that the motive that had been suggested in the first instance had been conclusively proved to have existed in this case. His learned friend had taken up the motive suggested in the middle or towards the end, but had ignored the first part of the motive set up. For the defence it was said that the motive suggested was that Hall would have obtained a certain amount of benefit under deeds. But that was only part of the motive suggested. What was the motive? To discover that they must go to first causes. It had been proved that for a series of years the prisoner had been committing forgeries, falsifying bank accounts, forging promissory notes, inducing the banker to discount them by pretending that they were ordinary business transactions. Was there no motive when the prisoner on the 9th of September 1885, four months before Captain Cain's death, gave a mortgage to his banker over 3000 acres of land in Southland, subject to a first mortgage of £4000 to one Allan Scott, and asked the banker not to register that mortgage, as it would affect his credit; and then taking advantage of the consideration of his banker and in fraud of that mortgage, he put a further mortgage for £3500, dated the 30th November, which virtually rendered the mortgage given to the bank valueless? Was not the fact of these things being in existence, with his forgeries coming due from time to time and being renewed as to part, and the knowledge that the deeds he had forged might be questioned at any time and brought in evidence against him, insufficient to supply evidence of motive? Were not these things urging the prisoner to do something to meet the difficulties in which he found himself involved? Although it might be the fact that the prisoner did allow his wife to sign the deed of covenant of the 5th of December, and that he might have influenced her not to sign it if he had been so minded, would that matter to the prisoner if he had determined to remove Captain Cain from his path so shortly afterwards? Could it be said that the act of the prisoner in allowing his wife without any demur to execute that deed is any answer to the motive suggested as existing from the financial difficulties and forgeries in which he was involved? The motive covered far wider grounds than the deeds of settlement referred to, and the advantage which the prisoner might have supposed he would obtain by Captain Cain's death covered also larger grounds than anything the deeds indicated. After Captain Cain's death it was found that his property only amounted to £3000; but it might well have been that the prisoner thought it would amount to a great deal more. Then it was surely no forced assumption on the part of the Crown that whatever Captain Cain had to leave would be divided between Hall's wife and Mrs Newton, Captain Cain's stepdaughters—or, at all events, that they would get the greater part of it; and that he did look forward to something of the kind they had most reliable evidence in the fact that Miss Gillon told them that when the prisoner was informed by his wife that Captain Cain had made another will, he was pleased with the intelligence and said, "All the better for us, Kitty." The prisoner might have entertained very large expectations, and therefore the learned counsel for the prisoner was wrong in saying that it was a motiveless murder, because the prisoner would not have gained anything by it. His learned friend had put it to the jury, "Can you believe that on such a motive this man should proceed to cruelly kill a dying man?" Those were the words of his learned friend, and he (Mr Haggitt) would say to them, Did this man hesitate to try to kill a dying woman? They had heard the story; it had came out fully in evidence before them. At a time when the prisoner's wife, one would think, should have had the greatest claim to his loving care; when she had just borne to him his first child, when she would naturally look for an increase of his love and care for her, what did they find? They found that on the fourth day after the birth of the child the prisoner commenced to poison his wife, and that he carried on this work systematically and regularly until his wife was reduced to such a state that she had to be kept up by injections. And yet, although this was the fact, although the only nourishment his wife got was a little ice-water in the mouth, and the only things that sustained her were injections, the prisoner managed with devilish ingenuity to poison the very ice-water she had to drink and to poison the brandy which was to go into her injection. And yet the learned counsel for the defence said in the face of such knowledge that they must not believe that on such a motive as the one suggested the prisoner proceeded cruelly to kill a dying man. If they believed the facts that had come out in evidence in this case, was there anything they could not believe the prisoner to be guilty of? Would they find it necessary to look for any considerable motive, or for any motive at all, in fact, to induce the prisoner to remove any man that stood in his road? That was the case which the Crown had made, and what was the defence—the answer made by his learned friends to meet the case. First there was the suggestion that deceased Captain Cain might have had Bright's disease and might have died from apoplexy. The jury would have to swallow that suggestion in the face of the evidence that symptoms of antimonial poisoning existed in Cain's lifetime and in the face of the fact that antimony was found in the body after death. In order to accept that suggestion they would have to come to the conclusion that Dr

Macintyre knew nothing whatever about his business; that he was not fit to act as a medical man, and that having his patient before him daily and watching the various stages of his illness, knew so little about his business that other medical men who simply listened to the symptoms were able to say that Bright's disease existed, while he was unable to discover any signs of it. But a further answer to this was that if this had been so no antimony would have been found after death. If death was the result of uremic poisoning and of Bright's disease, how was the antimony accounted for? That was the poser which he had put to the medical men called for the defence, and, with the notable exception of Dr Bakewell, they were all unable to account for the antimony being there, except on the supposition that the symptoms exhibited were the result of, or their severity was increased by, the antimony found. That was the first defence set up. The next defence was that Dr Ogston performed a slovenly post mortem. What on earth had that to do with it. Even supposing it to be the case, and the learned Crown prosecutor denied that it was so, what on earth had that to do with the case? They should recollect that the circumstances of the case were peculiar. This was not the case of an inquest to ascertain the cause of death. The man's death was supposed to be accounted for by natural causes, and he had been buried eight months before circumstances arose which rendered Dr Macintyre doubtful as to whether the death had been a natural one or a foul one. Then the corpse was disinterred not for the purpose of examining the kidneys and the heart and brain, but for the purpose of ascertaining whether the suspicions that had occurred to Dr Macintyre were well founded or not. The examination was mainly to ascertain whether there was antimony in the body. It was a post mortem out of the ordinary run altogether, and what had Dr Ogston done or neglected to do for which the learned counsel for the accused had attempted to scarify him? All that could be said was that he had omitted to take notes, and it was a matter which rested entirely with himself whether he should do that or not. Certain books had been referred to which advised that a certain course should be taken at post mortem examinations, but nobody was bound by those opinions, and they did not affect the case in the slightest degree. Did the learned counsel for the defence mean to say that Dr Ogston had told deliberate untruths? No. All that was said was that he had not taken notes, and the result was simply that he had to give his evidence from memory, and he had given his evidence without hesitation and without qualification. He (the learned Crown prosecutor) had not made notes, though perhaps he ought to have done so—they did not always do what they ought to,—and it appeared to him that the attack which had been made upon Dr Ogston was utterly and entirely unjustified by any circumstances which had occurred in court. The next suggestion for the defence was that the whole motive suggested had not been proved, but with that he had dealt already. Then it was suggested that the prisoner could not have poisoned the bottles upon the table, because he might have been seen putting the poison into the medicine and other things. The next thing was that there was a certain amount of mystery about this household. He (the learned counsel for the Crown) did not know what to make of that, and he did not think his learned friend had made much of it. The next thing was that the Crown did not call Buchanan, Hibbard, or Newton. Well the Crown did not call Newton because Newton was not to be found, and if the Crown did not call Buchanan and Hibbard, the defence had called both. As to the evidence given by these witnesses, Hibbard had proved a fact they were not aware of before, namely, that the prisoner had a book on poisons in his possession two years before it was thought he had such a book ; and Buchanan, who had declined to give evidence for the Crown, had given evidence entirely at variance with all the other evidence before the jury. The only other point for the defence was that the jury ought to be frightened of making a mistake, because mistakes had been made by juries previously. As against these points for the defence, the Crown had made out this case:—First, it was proved that the prisoner was a poisoner, and that even his own wife was not safe from being one of his victims ; next, that he had studied antimony for years of his life; 3rd, that he was in difficulties, a forger of promissory notes and land mortgages, and fraudulently giving a mortgage on property previously mortgaged to a banker; next, that he had antimony in his possession, the possession of which he was unable to account for on any reasonable theory ; 6th, that he was in constant attendance on Cain ; 7th, that he had expectations from Cain's death; 8th, that the commencement of his attendance upon Cain was the commencement of the continued symptoms of antimonial poisoning; 9th, the fact that antimony was found in the body; 10th, that after Cain's death the prisoner, who had been waiting for his house, took possession of and occupied it. In addition to these they would find nothing to suggest suicide ; nor any suspicion even that anyone else had an interest in administering poison, or had poison in possession to administer ; and that there was no other reasonable way of accounting for the death, and that it had been caused by antimonial poisoning. It had been said that of all forms of death the most detestable was that of death by poisoning, because it was of all others the most difficult to prevent by manhood or forethought and was most difficult to detect, for the suspicion of it was so abhorrent to right-minded people that with the evidence of it before them people could not bring themselves to believe that people apparently friendly with their victim were actually poisoning him. Comment had been made on the small quantity of poison found in the body, and it was said that the whole amount as had been determined by quantitative

analysis was unsufficient to account for death. Now it would be most unreasonable, and would lead to the grossest injustice and to impunity in the very worst of crimes, to require that the effect of poisoning should be proved by any special and exclusive means. Every case must depend upon its own particular circumstances and must be proved by the best evidence which could be adduced, and by such an amount of relevant facts, whether direct or circumstantial, as would establish the imputed guilt to a moral certainty and to the exclusion of any other reasonable hypothesis. That, he submitted, had been the case here, and if it was a moral certainty to their minds that this crime, difficult as it was to prove, had been traced home to the prisoner, they would know what their duty was. The same duty did not devolve upon him as devolved upon the prisoner's advocate ; his position was merely an official one, and he had somewhat of the same kind of duty to perform as the jury. And his duty was equally as unpleasant to him as their duty would be to them. It was, however, a necessity of the situation that someone should prosecute, and it was a necessity that others should constitute the jury to hear and decide upon the evidence. He had done his duty to the best of his ability, and it would now remain for the jury to do theirs after hearing what his Honor had to say.

His Honor, in summing up, said : Gentlemen of the jury,—The prisoner is indicted for the wilful murder of Henry Cain. The case which has come before you has practically resolved itself into this : that the accused is charged with accelerating the death of Henry Cain by the administration of antimony. Now, if it be the case that the accused, by wilfully administering antimony, has accelerated even in the slightest degree the death of Cain, it will be your duty to find him guilty upon the present indictment. The case, as has been put to you, may be properly divided into two branches, each one of which is independent of the other. The first question is whether the death of Cain was accelerated by the administration of antimony. The second question is whether that antimony was administered by the prisoner Hall. The two questions are, as I have said, really independent one of the other, though the evidence as to both questions is inevitably connected to a certain extent. I will take the two branches of the case separately, and will first consider and lay before you the evidence on the point as to whether the death of Cain was accelerated by antimony. Of that you must be satisfied affirmatively. You must be satisfied beyond all reasonable doubt that the death was so accelerated, and that there is no other reasonable way of accounting for the death ; or, to put it in another way, as put by Mr Chapman fairly enough : you have to be satisfied that had it not been for the administration of antimony the deceased would not have died at the point of time at which he did ; that he would have lived longer. Now the case the Crown have endeavoured to make out on this branch is shortly as follows :—Cain was suffering from a very lowering and wasting disease ; antimony is a powerul depressent, and would tend to aggravate the action of the disease. Therefore the necessary action of the administration of antimony would be in such a case to accelerate and precipitate the termination, which in the natural order of things would occur later. The case for Crown could, perhaps, be put by an illustration, though I need hardly tell you that no illustration, however plausible it may seem, can safely be relied on. You have, of course, seen a locomotive engine in the process of shunting a truck. The engine gives to the truck a certain impetus. The truck, therefore, is impelled by a certain initial velocity, but from the moment of impact there are several forces tending to bring the truck to a standstill: gravitation, resistance of the atmosphere, and friction. After a certain time and at a certain point if the line is level the truck will come to a standstill. If there is somebody in the truck who puts on a brake it will come to a standstill sooner. Now that may be taken as an illustration of Captain Cain's case as the Crown has asked you to look at it. They say the wheels of Captain Cain's life were going slower and slower, and would have come to a standstill at no distant point in any case, but that the administration of antimony was pretically in the nature of putting on a brake or something of that kind, which from the nature of things would make the wheels stop at an earlier period. On the part of the defence it has been suggested that this case is not satisfactorily made out, and that there are other reasonable hypotheses which would account for the death; and, notably, it was suggested that a reasonable way of accounting for the death was that it might have been occasioned by uremic poisoning, or by effusion of blood on the brain, and that either of these causes might happen altogether independently of the administartion of antimony. I propose, as I have said, to bring the evidence on this part of the case before you first. The evidence divides itself into two parts—the phenomena which were observed, and the inferences which the various skilled witnesses drew from these phenomena. I am afraid it is impossible in considering the evidence first to take the phenomena and then the inferences. It would be the clearest way of putting it, but there is such a mass of evidence that I think I should have some difficulty in doing so. I am afraid we shall have to discuss the phenomena and the inferences which the doctors draw—at any rate to some extent—together. While on this point I might just as well point out to you the distinction in the nature of the evidence of experts, especially between what they have seen and evidence of the conclusions they arrive at from their observations. You have to look at the inferential evidence of experts with considerably greater caution, and to weigh it more carefully than you have to weigh the evidence of the facts which they say they have seen themselves. [His Honor here proceeded to review the evidence with regard to the appearances Captain Cain presented in his life, and also the *post mortem* appearances, reading and commenting upon extracts from the evidence of the medical men, and of the witnesses who had

attended Captain Cain during his illness. Referring in the course of his comments to Dr Ogston's evidence, his Honor said that notes of course should have been taken in any such case; but it came to this, he did not take them at the time, and some few days afterwards he did, but from circumstances not under the control of the court those notes were missing. So Dr Ogston had really to rely on his memory, but he spoke mainly to broad facts.] His Honor then continued as follows: — The next branch of the inquiry is whether the antimony found in the body was administered by the prisoner. Antimony, as you have heard, is not a natural part of the body, and it must have been administered during life, and probably in solution, and the most ordinary form in which it is found in solution is tartar emetic. How, then, did this antimony come there? You will of course have to be satisfied beyond all reasonable doubt that its presence was not the result of accident. We know Dr Macintyre never prescribed antimony, and the only possible suggestion of accident is with regard to that bottle of cough mixture which was bought on January 14, and the contents of which were not known. It was not part of Dr Macintyre's prescription, and the witness Gunn said that in all patent cough mixtures there is either antimony or ipecacuanha wine. But we have evidence that antimony is very little used, and although put down to him it does not seem that the bottle was for him, or that his attendants ever had the recollection of administering anything but the cough mixture and things Dr Macintyre prescribed. During the last 14 days of his life we know that Cain was bedridden ; so that he could not have got up and administered the antimony to himself. I mention these things because it is necessary for you to be reasonably satisfied that it was not by accident and that Cain did not take it of his own accord. Then how is the prisoner connected with the administration of the antimony? I need hardly say it is not sufficient to show that Cain did not take it of his own accord, and that it was not accidentally administered, and that the prisoner, amongst a number of other persons, had an opportunity of doing it. You want more than that to connect the prisoner with the transaction. The first thing we hear of him in connection with poison is that he had "Taylor on Poisons" some time in 1884. He was suffering from sciatica, neuralgia, and asthma, and possessed himself of this book. Then we have the evidence of Hutton as to his buying another copy, according to him, in June and also referring to Headland's book on the Action of Medicines, especially inquiring about antimony. This was before he made friends with Cain, and he seems also to have spoken about antimony for use in cigarettes for asthma. Dr Ogston seems to think it impossible that antimony could be used in cigarettes, but there is another reference to a book in which arseniate of antimony is spoken of as used in cigarettes for asthma. Anyhow, we know that early in the year the prisoner had the book on poisons, and a considerable quantity of antimony—two drachms. Later in the year 1885 he bought some atropia and wine of colchicum—the atropia on two occasions, and the colchicum on one. But I need hardly say these do not enter into this case seriously, as they must form matter of mere speculation. There we find the prisoner had numerous opportunities of access to Cain. He became friendly to him some time in November, and called pretty often then. He sat up with him twice, on Christmas Eve and the night before, and Miss Houston took the latter part of the night. Miss Houston did not observe that he was sick after Hall had sat up with him, although on Christmas Day he was very sick indeed. I have gone through the evidence to show that before he made it up with Cain the latter was sick, and I have pointed to the prescription of the 3rd November for nausea, and to the fact that at the end of November or beginning of December Cain used to complain of his whisky. Hall did not stay at the house, and the whisky was not kept for Cain alone. He was a hospitable man, so I suppose other people would have suffered unless Hall could have been present. Then after this Hall's visits became more constant; he stayed for a few minutes every morning, and the sickness seemed to continue. There is no evidence of any particular drink administered by Hall that Cain was sick after, except on that occasion at lunch spoken of by Mrs Ostler. The sickness seems to have come on at night, irrespective of the presence of Hall. All that can be said, therefore, is that Hall if he had been inclined to poison Cain had at this time plenty of opportunity for doing so, and that other people had the same opportunity. If a man lays himself out to poison a sick man, and has constant access, his most likely course to avert danger would be to put it into his physic, not in liquor which was on the table and open to anyone. Hall might do this, so might anyone else who had an interest in poisoning Cain; and it seems to me to be on the whole a question of saying that Hall had an opportunity of doing it and therefore he did it. Up to this point, then, the chief evidence against Hall seems to be his possession of the book "Taylor on Poisons" and of these poisons. It was correctly said by the counsel for the Crown that it is not necessary to prove motive; but at the same time, where there is a doubt whether a particular crime was committed by a particular man, the fact that he had a motive is very properly dwelt upon. Now, in this case my motive suggested is that Hall was in want of money, and that Cain's death would bring him money. And I think it may very well be taken that he was in want of money, because a man does not fortify his banking account with forgeries and undertake transactions like that of the mortgage unless he is in a very bad way. The question is therefore whether there is reasonable evidence that Cain's death would put money into Hall's pocket. Mrs Hall was interested in two settlements, and as to one of these, Mrs Newton, her sister, was also interested. In the first—that in which both were interested—the parties on 5th December made a deed which gave Cain an annuity of £300 a year and the use of Woodlands during his life. Had it not been for the execution of that deed, Cain's death would not, so far as this

settlement was concerned, have been of the least benefit to Mrs Hall. She had a life interest in the property wholly independent of Cain, and by this deed they granted Cain the annuity and use of the house. The deed was dated December 5, and Mr Knubbley, the solicitor, says it was executed by Mrs Hall with her husband's full consent and knowledge. All that Mrs Hall seems to have had under the settlement was a life interest in the property, subsequently transferable to her children, but she deprived herself of her life interest in part of the annuity and also of the proceeds of Woodlands. She also seems by this deed to have had some claim against Cain, because he had advanced sums to Mrs Newton for a larger amount than she was entitled to. Therefore it was suggested by the defence that it is absurd to suppose a man would voluntarily allow his wife to execute a deed giving Cain a life interest under the settlement if he intended to get rid of him. A simpler way would have been to tell his wife not to sign it. Then there was another settlement under which Mrs Hall had a life interest in certain property, and had given herself a disposing power of it by will only so that she could not deal with the *corpus*. Hall wanted to cancel this—of course for the purpose of getting the money. Le Cren said in December that Cain objected to this, and I confess it struck me on reading the affidavit produced, and I said so at the time: "Here was a strong motive on Hall's part for getting rid of Cain, and yet we have an affidavit sworn by Cain to Knubbley showing that he (Cain) was at that time quite satisfied that what Hall wanted should be done, and a friendly suit begun." So it seems that Hall was a party to a friendly suit with his wife for the purpose of getting rid of the trust, when at that time he could have got all he wanted without any trouble. Then the third thing it is suggested that Hall would get by Cain's death was something under his will. There is evidence that Hall was aware that a new will had been made, but it was suggested as inconsistent that he, as a party to the deed of December 5, could have supposed that Cain had any large property to leave. Further, there were his daughters, who were not blood relations, and a nephew who was, of whom he seemed to have been fond. I have dealt now with matters up to Captain Cain's death; but there is certain evidence which has been admitted and which you have a perfect right to take into consideration and give every reasonable influence to in considering the question as to whether antimony was administered by Hall. Of course I allude to the evidence you have before you that a few months later his wife was ill. There were symptoms of antimony observed in her for a considerable time by Dr Macintyre, and ultimately liquids received from Hall for her were seized and found themselves to contain antimony, and antimony was also found upon Hall. You have a perfect right to take all these circumstances into account in considering how antimony got into Captain Cain's body. If antimony is found in the body of a person to whom the accused has constant access, and if later antimony was without doubt administered by him to another person, it is for you to say if it is not a reasonable conclusion that the antimony found in the body of the person first named was also administered by the prisoner. You have no business at all to go beyond the evidence before you, but it is your duty to make any use of that which seems reasonable, and to draw any inference from it as to the administration of antimony by the prisoner to Cain that you may think it justifies. It seems to me to be perfectly clear that this is the key to the whole thing connecting the prisoner with it. You need not be in the least afraid to act upon it if you think it justifiable, because it seems to me the real key of the position, and in the event of a conviction I shall reserve the point as to the propriety of this admission for the Court of Appeal. However, the evidence is before you and you can deal with it just as you please; and it is your duty to draw any reasonable inference from it that can be drawn. I do not know that I need say any more. You have, as I say, to be satisfied beyond all reasonable doubt—to the exclusion of any rational hypothesis—of two things: firstly, that Cain's death was accelerated by antimony to some degree, however slight; secondly, that that antimony was wilfully administered by the prisoner. You have displayed singular attention and patience, gentlemen, with respect to this case. and I have no doubt at all that you will consider the evidence carefully and form your conclusion. You will now please consider your verdict, gentlemen.

The jury retired at 6.20 p.m.

THE VERDICT—"GUILTY."

The jury returned to the court at 7.45 p.m.

The Registrar: Gentlemen, are you agreed upon your verdict?

The Foreman: Yes.

The Registrar: How say you, gentlemen, do you find the prisoner "Guilty" or "Not guilty"?

The Foreman: "Guilty."

His Honor: As I have already intimated, it is my intention to reserve for the opinion of the Court of Appeal the question as to the admissibility of the evidence which was objected to by

the counsel for the prisoner. Under these circumstances the Court of Appeal Act gives me the alternative either of postponing to pass sentence or to pass sentence now and to respite execution. I shall have the opportunity hereafter of giving more fully the reasons, which I have already to some extent given, why this point should be reserved. I think on the whole it would be more convenient in the interests of justice if the sentence were passed now and execution is respited until the decision of the Court of Appeal upon the point can be had.

THE SENTENCE—"DEATH."

His Honor: Will you call upon the prisoner, Mr Gordon.

The Registrar; Prisoner, have you anything to say why the sentence of the court should not be passed upon you?

The Prisoner: I do not see that it will do any good.

His Honor in passing sentence said: As I have already intimated to you, prisoner, the legal question connected with your case will be considered by the Court of Appeal. If there is anything in the point you will have the benefit of it. I do not think it is in the least necessary for me, whatever may be the ultimate result of the point which is now reserved, to add one word to the sentence which by law I have to pronounce. (His Honor, assuming the black cap, continued): The judgment of the law is that you, Thomas Hall, be taken from the place where you now are to the prison from whence you came, and thence to the place of execution, and that there, in manner and form by law appointed, you be hanged by the neck until you are dead. The prisoner can be removed.

The prisoner having been removed,

His Honor, addressing the jury, said: I have to thank you, gentlemen, for the very great patience you have exhibited during this long protracted case. If it is any satisfaction to you, I can only say that if the evidence to which I have referred is properly evidence in the case, I think you are justified in the conclusion at which you have arrived. I have to thank you, gentlemen, on behalf of the colony for your services.

The jury were discharged, and the court rose at 8.15 p.m.

www.ingramcontent.com/pod-product-compliance
Lightning Source LLC
Chambersburg PA
CBHW020334090426
42735CB00009B/1538